THE
EVERYTHING
GUIDE TO THE
AUTOIMMUNE DIET

Dear Reader,

As a child growing up in the era of astronauts and moon landings of the 1960s, I was swept up in the idea of exploring space and strange new worlds. As those dreams gave way to reality, I found myself following in my grandmother's and father's footsteps by becoming a chiropractor instead.

After graduation, I found the idea of just adjusting patients on a daily basis to be too boring for my adventurous spirit and began studying every aspect of health and holistic healthcare. My father's subsequent illness and passing became the rocket fuel for going beyond the bounds of modern and holistic medicine, and understanding health and sickness in expansive ways. As my knowledge base grew, my patients became even more complex, constantly challenging me to go even further in my understanding. In today's world, we all share the same fate. We live in a time in which the daily stresses of life and the burdens of toxicity are rapidly exceeding our ability to adapt and cope, often leading to a life of chronic inflammation and eventual disease.

This book provides a way to survive and thrive while creating a life of health and vitality.

Here's to your health!

Jeffrey S. McCombs, DC

Welcome to the EVERYTHING® Series!

These handy, accessible books give you all you need to tackle a difficult project, gain a new hobby, comprehend a fascinating topic, prepare for an exam, or even brush up on something you learned back in school but have since forgotten.

You can choose to read an Everything® book from cover to cover or just pick out the information you want from our four useful boxes: e-questions, e-facts, e-alerts, and e-ssentials.

We give you everything you need to know on the subject, but throw in a lot of fun stuff along the way, too.

We now have more than 400 Everything® books in print, spanning such wide-ranging categories as weddings, pregnancy, cooking, music instruction, foreign language, crafts, pets, New Age, and so much more. When you're done reading them all, you can finally say you know Everything®!

QUESTION

Answers to common questions

FACT

Important snippets of information

ALERT

Urgent warnings

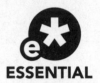

ESSENTIAL

Quick handy tips

PUBLISHER Karen Cooper

MANAGING EDITOR, EVERYTHING® SERIES Lisa Laing

COPY CHIEF Casey Ebert

ASSISTANT PRODUCTION EDITOR Alex Guarco

ACQUISITIONS EDITOR Hillary Thompson

SENIOR DEVELOPMENT EDITOR Brett Palana-Shanahan

EVERYTHING® SERIES COVER DESIGNER Erin Alexander

Visit the entire Everything® series at *www.everything.com*

THE EVERYTHING®

GUIDE TO THE
AUTOIMMUNE
DIET

Restore your immune system and manage chronic illness
with healing, nourishing foods

Dr. Jeffrey McCombs, DC

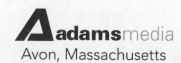

Avon, Massachusetts

To John-Roger and the love that lifts us all.

An Everything® Series Book.
Everything® and everything.com® are registered trademarks of F+W Media, Inc.

Published by
Adams Media, a division of F+W Media, Inc.
57 Littlefield Street, Avon, MA 02322. U.S.A.
www.adamsmedia.com

ISBN 10: 1-4405-8732-9
ISBN 13: 978-1-4405-8732-0
eISBN 10: 1-4405-8733-7
eISBN 13: 978-1-4405-8733-7

Printed in the United States of America.

10   9   8   7   6   5   4   3   2   1

Library of Congress Cataloging-in-Publication Data

McCombs, Jeffrey, author.
    The everything guide to the autoimmune diet / Jeffrey McCombs.
        p. cm. -- (Everything series book)
    Includes index.
    ISBN 978-1-4405-8732-0 (pb) -- ISBN 1-4405-8732-9 (pb) -- ISBN 978-1-4405-8733-7 (ebook)
-- ISBN 1-4405-8733-7 (ebook)
    I. Title. II. Series: Everything series.
    [DNLM: 1. Autoimmune Diseases--diet therapy--Cookbooks. 2. Autoimmune Diseases--
diet therapy--Popular Works. 3. Cooking--methods. WD 305]
    RC600
    616.97'80654--dc23
                        2015006172

Always follow safety and commonsense cooking protocol while using kitchen utensils, operating ovens and stoves, and handling uncooked food. If children are assisting in the preparation of any recipe, they should always be supervised by an adult.

Cover image © iStockphoto.com/AR-tem.

This book is available at quantity discounts for bulk purchases.
For information, please call 1-800-289-0963.

Contents

Introduction **9**

01 What Is Autoimmune Disease? / 11

Defining Autoimmune Disease **12**

A Brief History **14**

Autoimmune Conditions **16**

Who Is at Risk? **19**

What to Expect with a Diagnosis **22**

02 The Enemy Within / 27

Distinguishing the Body's Cells: Self versus Non-Self **28**

The Immune System's Toolbox **31**

Friend or Foe? Immune System Responses **39**

Worm Food: Helminthic Therapy Research **42**

03 The Environmental Impact / 45

Is It Your Environment or Your Genetics? **46**

Toxins Are Passed from Mother to Child **49**

The Burden of Environmental Toxins **53**

Unique Problems Humans Face **56**

04 A Difficult Diagnosis / 59

When a Wrong Diagnosis Occurs **60**

Misunderstood Autoimmune Conditions **66**

How Autoimmune Treatments Can Worsen Your Condition **67**

Chasing Symptoms Instead of the Cause **69**

Spontaneous Remission: When Unexpected Improvement Occurs **72**

05 Mindful Steps for Healing / 75

Common Medical Mistakes in Treating Autoimmune Disease **76**

The Mind-Body Connection in Autoimmunity **81**

Meditation, Prayer, and Mindfulness **84**

Resolving Stress, Tension, and Trauma **86**

06 Antibiotics, Candida, and the Gut / 91

Antibiotics: Both Cure and Curse **92**

Antibiotics and LPS **95**

Candida-Related Conditions **97**

Inflammation and Candida **99**

Maintaining Good Gut Health **101**

07 **Natural Solutions / 105**

Vitamins **106**

Minerals **115**

Herbs **117**

Getting Healthy with Dirt: The Hygiene Hypothesis **120**

08 **The Autoimmune Diet / 123**

Cooling the Fires with Gluten-Free Foods **124**

How the Autoimmune Diet Works **124**

Nature's Answers **127**

Detoxifying Your Meals **129**

Juicing and Cleanses **133**

Autoimmune Yes and No Foods **135**

09 **Functional Cooking / 139**

Adopting a Gluten-Free Lifestyle **140**

Low-Histamine Foods **143**

Resistant Starches **145**

The Secrets of Spices **146**

Meal Planning for Long-Term Health **148**

A New Beginning **149**

10 **Breakfast / 151**

11 **Lunch / 165**

12 **Dinner / 181**

13 **Sauces and Marinades / 195**

14 **Soups and Stews / 205**

15 **Salads / 221**

16 **Vegetables / 235**

17 **Snacks / 251**

18 **Beverages / 265**

19 **Juicing / 271**

Appendix A: Resources **281**

Appendix B: Sample Meal Plans **285**

Index **293**

Acknowledgments

First, I'd like to thank all the patients whom I have been privileged to serve and assist during the course of my 30-plus years of practice since 1984. It has been their willingness and patience—combined with a sincere yearning to know more, do better, and live a longer, healthier life—that has helped fuel my desire to assist them. Each of them has taught me to dig deeper, learn more, and go beyond the known and into the unknown to find the answers that they and so many others need. It is often through a willingness to abandon the safety of the known in order to discover new frontiers that a doctor finds the answers to the puzzles of imbalance that are reflected in disease. A doctor is forever a student to the patient.

I'd like to thank Adams Media for the opportunity to once again share the wealth of information that I have gathered during my years of practice as a doctor of chiropractic.

Thanks go out to Faith Kincaid for sharing with us her juice recipes while preparing for delivery of her baby girl, Stella. A huge thank-you to Hugo Alvarado for creating all the wonderful food recipes in this book. There must be a restaurant business in this somewhere for you, or perhaps, your own book? Thanks again to Hugo, as well as Blanca Dominguez for holding down the office while I researched and wrote this book.

Thanks to my father, who held out the example of what a true doctor can be, and my mom, who taught me to reach for the stars. Love to my siblings—Kim, Kelly, and Terry—for their lifelong support and love.

Loving thanks to Ana Maria and our children, Ethan and Ana Sophia. Two books in the period of a year is too much time for "Papi" to be away from both his family and fatherly duties. Your love makes it all possible. Time to play now.

Introduction

THE FIELD OF AUTOIMMUNE science is rapidly evolving and ever changing. In fact, to say that there is a field at all at this point is still somewhat premature. Autoimmunity is currently divided among many different specialties, while one unifying theory is being birthed into existence by a few brave researchers. Until this new field is born, many people will have to wander about an uncharted map of autoimmunity searching for the answer to their dilemma.

Autoimmunity is like one of the earliest maps of the planet. Every country knows who they are, yet they know little about all the others. What is known of the world of autoimmunity is a loosely identified map of where everyone is, without knowing how they are all connected.

Once someone is diagnosed with an autoimmune condition, he will often wander about this map and have a greater chance of ending up in another country, representative of yet another autoimmune diagnosis. Having an autoimmune condition predisposes one to having another. This alone is evidence of an underlying connection between them.

Whether you have one autoimmune diagnosis, two, or more, the diagnosis is only the beginning point. Learning how to manage the condition and correcting the imbalances that created it will be where all your time and effort is spent. Modern medicine believes that there are no cures for autoimmune diseases, yet more and more people are finding that there are ways to reverse autoimmune diseases and science supports these approaches.

While many traditional medical doctors will only provide medications to suppress symptoms, there is another course of action. Holistic doctors and practitioners view illness and disease as a symptom of a life that is out of balance. Using natural approaches such as vitamins, minerals, herbs, homeopathy, diet, meditation, exercise, lifestyle changes, and more, they identify where the imbalances are and work with the patients to help bring their lives back into balance. In this approach, the patient is the most important key to the success, or cure.

Each approach in holistic medicine is like a suit that needs to be custom tailored to each person. What works for one person may not work for another. One person may have dietary restrictions that another person does not require. General principles will apply across the board, much like the untailored suit, but individual adjustments may have to be made in order to determine the best fit.

To determine what works best for each person can take time. It helps to be patient in this process, as it is an evolving process of discovery. For those who insist on an easy, take-a-pill approach, traditional medicine is their answer, even though that branch of medicine has already stated that it has no answers to autoimmunity. For those who are willing to follow the longer path that supplies answers and results, holistic medicine is their path.

Although this is a book for autoimmune conditions, it has applications for every condition, as every autoimmune condition is based in inflammation and inflammation is a part of every condition. If you have a cold, this book can help you. If you have cancer, this book can help you. It is not a cure-all; it is a tool to put in your toolbox to build a life of health.

CHAPTER 1

What Is Autoimmune Disease?

The body's immune system is a powerful shield that protects the body against foreign invaders, toxins, and abnormal processes that can lead to sickness and disease. The health of the immune system is often seen as a measure of the overall health of the body. When that same immune response turns on the body and starts attacking its own cells and tissues, however, these powerful processes can initiate a cascade of effects that become the cause of sickness and disease in the body. What results is known as autoimmune disease.

Defining Autoimmune Disease

Autoimmune disease is commonly defined as the process by which the body's immune system attacks the body's own cells and tissues. The current understanding of autoimmunity views this self-attack as a mistake that the immune system is making. By attacking healthy tissues, the immune system creates a disease process, as opposed to protecting the body against disease. The immune system is a great protector. It protects you against all types of problematic microbes that are foreign to the body. It also helps protect you against the microbes normally found on your skin and in your body. In this role, it is also the great regulator, and even sometimes the trash collector, when toxins become backed up within the body. When imbalances have gone too far and cancer cells start to develop, it is the immune system's responsibility to break down the tumor cells and stop the cancer process. In order to play a variety of roles, the immune system has a tremendous complexity that enables it to meet almost any challenge.

FACT

Our understanding of the immune system is constantly evolving. Since the 1960s, each decade has seen major advances in our understanding of the immune system, and we are still a long way off from being able to describe everything that takes place. How this system functions with every other system, organ, and cell of the body is still poorly understood.

The complexity of the immune system is something that science continues to unravel and discover. Limitations in our ability to perceive exactly what is taking place puts science in a position to make interpretations of what they find and then draw conclusions based on a generally accepted consensus as to what it all means. What's true today may not be true tomorrow, or it may only be the tip of the iceberg in an ongoing journey of discovery. That tip of the iceberg, however, fills volumes of textbooks, so hopefully a simplified version is enough to gain a little bit better understanding of what's taking place.

Nonspecific Immunity

One of the very first immune responses is one that is designated as a nonspecific response. The nonspecific immune response is also called the innate response. Immune cells are always circulating throughout the body ready to identify anything that is not normally present in the body and attempt to eliminate it by consuming it and destroying it. Cells that perform this type of function are various white blood cells like macrophages, neutrophils, dendritic cells, NK cells, and other substances. Each of these cells can play a role in autoimmune diseases when the immune system is not being regulated properly or there are conditions present that suppress the function of some cells while boosting the function of others. Balance is always an important key to health on all levels.

Specific Immunity

Specific immunity is a response that is more targeted and based on the immune system operating on specific information about what needs to be done. This response is also known as the adaptive response and comes into play when any substance is able to get past the innate immune response. When this happens, the alarm sounds and white blood cells known as B cells and T cells become activated. The B cells make up the body's humoral response and the T cells are a part of the body's cell-mediated response.

Cell-Mediated Response

The cell-mediated response involves white blood cells called thymus cells, or T cells. These cells are manufactured in the bone marrow and mature in the immune system's thymus gland. There are various T cells that normally work together in a coordinated fashion to help identify and eliminate intruders, as well as regulate the activity of other immune responses. Some of the major cells involved include Th1, Th2, Th17, Tregs, and the newly discovered ThGM cells. Some T cells help collect pieces of the intruders that were destroyed by the cells of the body's innate immune response. They present these pieces to the B cells, which can then develop a more specific and speedier immune response.

Humoral Response

The word *humoral* refers to the fluids of the body. When problematic foreign microbes, also known as pathogens, make it into the fluid spaces between cells without being stopped, the body's humoral response begins. The humoral response involves the deployment of white blood cells known as B cells. B cells are made in the bone marrow to arrest the invaders and stop any further advancement. The hallmark of the B cells is the production of antibodies, also known as immunoglobulins. The antibody is a sugar/protein combination produced by the B cells when the immune system recognizes harmful substances. These antibody substances aid in identifying and triggering other white blood cells to aid in the process of eliminating foreign substances. Once this process has been engaged, the body is able to remember and respond much faster should the same pathogen or substance enter the body again.

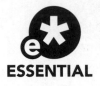

ESSENTIAL

In ancient Greece, the planetary elements of air, water, fire, and earth were understood to be represented in the body as blood, phlegm, yellow bile, and black bile, respectively. Imbalances between them, or impurities of these fluids in the body, were thought to result in disease. Modern medicine has abandoned this understanding of the body, while some holistic therapies continue to consider it.

As with everything else in the body, there is a great deal of cross-talk and cooperation between various immune cells and other cells of the body. It is a coordinated effort in which a symphony of players work together to produce the desired results. When all the notes are played at the right time for the right length at the right volume, it's a harmonious masterpiece. When there is discordance among the players, disastrous results can occur.

A Brief History

The history of autoimmune diseases is a rather loose-knit one. If you look at autoimmune conditions as one problem that spreads across many different parts of the body, you'd be more likely to establish a beginning point for the history of autoimmune diseases. Unfortunately, a cohesive approach to auto-immunity hasn't existed in medicine and only recently has the idea that auto-immunity is one field with multiple variations been suggested. Because the field of medicine is divided into many separate branches it hasn't allowed for easy associations between various autoimmune diseases.

For example, in the past, the rheumatologist specialized in autoim-mune joint and connective tissue problems, the gastroenterologist treated autoimmune conditions of the gut, and the neurologist treated autoimmune diseases of the nervous system. Each specialty was treating autoimmune diseases from the perspective of its individual specialty without considering them as a collective field.

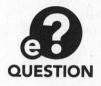

QUESTION

Can my cats and dogs also have an autoimmune condition?
Yes, rheumatoid arthritis, systemic lupus, anemia, and pemphigus are autoimmune conditions in humans that can show up in pets as well. Autoimmune conditions are not known to be transmissible between you and your pets, though, so don't worry about that. Some of the earliest findings of arthritis are from excavations of dinosaurs.

Rheumatoid arthritis (RA) has a history dating back thousands of years. The first formal description of RA was in the year 1800, when a French physi-cian, Augustin Jacob Landré-Beauvais, described it. Prior to that, the condi-tion can be seen in paintings that date back at least another hundred years or more. One early text from the year 123 described symptoms that are very similar to what we now know as rheumatoid arthritis and some excavations have found RA in the joints of humans from 4500 B.C.

The understanding of the body's immune system as being responsible for attacking itself was something that didn't exist until the mid-1960s. Subse-quent decades of research have created a large body of data that indicates that these various diseases can all be classified under one heading, replac-ing the fragmented medical approach of the past.

Autoimmune Conditions

There are over 150 autoimmune conditions in the body. The autoimmune response can affect every organ system of the body. According to the American Autoimmune Related Diseases Association (AARDA), there are approximately 50 million Americans suffering from autoimmune diseases. Worldwide those numbers increase, but sufferers tend to be predominantly located in developed countries, giving some indication that autoimmune diseases are a result of modern societies and all that goes with them.

FACT

Typically, a disease is considered autoimmune when it meets the criteria of Witebsky's postulates. Created by Ernst Witebsky in 1957, the four postulates include direct evidence of the presence of antibodies, indirect evidence from animal studies, circumstantial clinical evidence, and the presence of genetics that are similar to other autoimmune diseases.

According to the AARDA, the list of autoimmune diseases continues to grow and includes the following conditions:

- Acute disseminated encephalomyelitis (ADEM)
- Acute necrotizing hemorrhagic leukoencephalitis
- Addison's disease
- Agammaglobulinemia
- Alopecia areata
- Amyloidosis
- Ankylosing spondylitis
- Anti-GBM/anti-TBM nephritis
- Antiphospholipid syndrome (APS)
- Autoimmune angioedema
- Autoimmune aplastic anemia
- Autoimmune dysautonomia

- Autoimmune hepatitis
- Autoimmune hyperlipidemia
- Autoimmune immunodeficiency
- Autoimmune inner ear disease (AIED)
- Autoimmune myocarditis
- Autoimmune oophoritis
- Autoimmune pancreatitis
- Autoimmune retinopathy
- Autoimmune thrombocytopenic purpura (ATP)
- Autoimmune thyroid disease
- Autoimmune urticaria
- Axonal and neuronal neuropathies
- Balo's disease

- Behcet's disease
- Bullous pemphigoid
- Cardiomyopathy
- Castleman disease
- Celiac disease
- Chagas disease
- Chronic fatigue syndrome
- Chronic inflammatory demyelinating poly-neuropathy (CIDP)
- Chronic recurrent multifocal ostomyelitis (CRMO)
- Churg-Strauss syndrome
- Cicatricial pemphigoid/benign mucosal pemphigoid
- Crohn's disease
- Cogan's syndrome
- Cold agglutinin disease
- Congenital heart block
- Coxsackie myocarditis
- CREST disease
- Essential mixed cryoglobulinemia
- Demyelinating neuropathies
- Dermatitis herpetiformis
- Dermatomyositis
- Devic's disease (neuromyelitis optica)
- Discoid lupus
- Dressler's syndrome
- Endometriosis
- Eosinophilic esophagitis
- Eosinophilic fascitis
- Erythema nodosum
- Experimental allergic encephalomyelitis
- Evans syndrome
- Fibromyalgia
- Fibrosing alveolitis
- Giant cell arteritis
- Giant cell myocarditis
- Glomerulonephritis
- Goodpasture's syndrome
- Granulomatosis with polyangiitis (GPA)
- Graves' disease
- Guillain-Barre syndrome
- Hashimoto's encephalitis
- Hashimoto's thyroiditis
- Hemolytic anemia
- Henoch-Schonlein purpura
- Herpes gestationis
- Hypogammaglobulinemia
- Idiopathic thrombocytopenic purpura (ITP)
- IgA nephropathy
- IgG4-related sclerosing disease
- Immunoregulatory lipoproteins
- Inclusion body myositis
- Interstitial cystitis
- Juvenile arthritis
- Juvenile diabetes (type 1 diabetes)
- Juvenile myositis
- Kawasaki disease
- Lambert-Eaton syndrome
- Leukocytoclastic vasculitis
- Lichen planus
- Ligneous conjunctivitis
- Linear IgA disease (LAD)
- Lupus (SLE)
- Lyme disease, chronic
- Meniere's disease
- Microscopic polyangiitis
- Mixed connective tissue disease (MCTD)
- Mooren's ulcer
- Mucha-Habermann disease
- Multiple sclerosis
- Myasthenia gravis

- Myositis
- Narcolepsy
- Neutropenia
- Ocular cicatricial pemphigoid
- Optic neuritis
- Palindromic rheumatism
- PANDAS (pediatric autoimmune neuropsychiatric disorders associated with streptococcus)
- Paraneoplastic cerebellar degeneration
- Paroxysmal nocturnal hemoglobinuria (PNH)
- Parry Romberg syndrome
- Parsonage-Turner syndrome
- Pars planitis (peripheral uveitis)
- Pemphigus
- Peripheral neuropathy
- Perivenous encephalomyelitis
- Pernicious anemia
- POEMS syndrome
- Polyarteritis nodosa
- Type 1, 2, and 3 autoimmune polyglandular syndromes
- Polymyalgia rheumatica
- Polymyositis
- Postmyocardial infarction syndrome
- Postpericardiotomy syndrome
- Progesterone dermatitis
- Primary biliary cirrhosis
- Primary sclerosing cholangitis
- Psoriasis
- Psoriatic arthritis
- Idiopathic pulmonary fibrosis
- Pyoderma gangrenosum
- Pure red cell aplasia
- Raynaud's phenomenon

- Reactive arthritis
- Reflex sympathetic dystrophy
- Reiter's syndrome
- Relapsing polychondritis
- Restless legs syndrome
- Retroperitoneal fibrosis
- Rheumatic fever
- Rheumatoid arthritis
- Sarcoidosis
- Schmidt's syndrome
- Scleritis
- Scleroderma
- Sjogren's syndrome
- Sperm and testicular autoimmunity
- Stiff person syndrome
- Subacute bacterial endocarditis (SBE)
- Susac's syndrome
- Sympathetic ophthalmia
- Takayasu's arteritis
- Temporal arteritis/Giant cell arteritis
- Thrombocytopenic purpura (TTP)
- Tolosa-Hunt syndrome
- Transverse myelitis
- Type 1 diabetes
- Ulcerative colitis
- Undifferentiated connective tissue disease (UCTD)
- Uveitis
- Vasculitis
- Vesiculobullous dermatitis
- Vitiligo

As one can easily see from this list of more than 150 autoimmune conditions, autoimmunity is something that can occur almost anywhere in the body. The immune system functions throughout the body in one form or another, and an imbalanced response can begin in any tissue. Understanding more about who is at risk is one way to better gauge one's susceptibility.

Who Is at Risk?

Given the wide variety of diseases and conditions that affect various tissues throughout the body, autoimmunity can strike anyone, at almost any age. If you live in a modern society in an industrialized country, your chances are increased. The number of diseases being identified as autoimmune in nature also appears to be increasing, so one can expect that the number of people being affected will increase as well. Autoimmunity is a fact of life and everyone has some degree of it at one time or another, but the body for the most part should resolve the imbalances and restore homeostasis. That being said, there are some risk patterns that have emerged from the data so far.

Women

Women, by and large, are more affected than men by autoimmune diseases. In women under the age of sixty-five, autoimmune diseases are one of the top ten causes of death. Women are 75 percent more likely to suffer from an autoimmune disease. One theory as to the cause of this difference is the effect of hormones like estrogen that have been shown to increase autoimmune responses. Pregnancy has also been shown to be another causative factor in the creation of autoimmune responses. In both instances, hormones play an important role.

Estrogen

Researchers at the University of Genoa's Department of Internal Medicine cite estrogens as an enhancer of autoimmune responses, while androgens and progesterone are immune suppressors. A group of researchers from Naples, Italy, also found that a progesterone deficiency was common in women with thyroid and ovarian autoimmune disease.

In some instances, occurrences of autoimmune diseases in women is high, as is the case with lupus erythematosus, in which ratios can be as high as 9:1 or 10:1 (women versus men). Rheumatoid arthritis on the other hand has a smaller ratio of 4:1.

Pregnancy

On one hand, pregnancy seems like a natural source of autoimmune responses. The fetus is a foreign tissue to a mother's body, so one would expect some type of autoimmune reaction to its presence. Nature, however, in her infinite wisdom, designed a woman's body to be able to regulate her immune responses so as not to cause the loss of a pregnancy. This shift is the reason why some women who have an autoimmune condition find that their symptoms go away during pregnancy, only to return later. This sort of rebound could also activate latent autoimmune conditions that haven't expressed themselves yet.

Genetics

Scientists have noticed that autoimmune diseases have a tendency to occur in familial patterns. In some instances, such as diabetes and lupus, subsequent generations may end up having the same condition. In other familial instances, autoimmune conditions can be present but the exact disease may vary from one family member to another. One family member may have rheumatoid arthritis and another may have multiple sclerosis, and yet another one may have something entirely different.

FACT

Geography may be another factor in autoimmune conditions. Autoimmune diabetes occurs at six times the frequency in Finland as compared to the neighboring Karelian Republic of Russia, even though they share a common genetic background. Different environments may activate autoimmunity in those with the same genetic background.

The Multiple Autoimmune Disease Genetics Consortium (MADGC) found common underlying genetic patterns among rheumatoid arthritis, systemic lupus erythematosus, and type 1 diabetes. Multiple sclerosis, on the other hand, appears to have a different disease process. Despite the appearance of common underlying traits or genes there is no simple and predictable pattern of inheritance.

Environment

Environmental influences are also common among family members. People raised in the same house with the same genetics share the same susceptibility to develop autoimmune diseases. The variability in body types, intestinal flora, gender, age, and resiliency toward stress can account for the variation in the diseases that they develop, or even whether a condition develops at all.

ALERT

The human body is like a sponge to its environment. It can absorb whatever toxins are present in the world around it. While avoiding all toxins may be impossible, reducing and eliminating as many exposures as possible is almost mandatory when healing autoimmune conditions. Take baby steps to make your home a place of repair and regeneration for your body.

To date, being able to predict that someone will or will not have an autoimmune disease is almost impossible. If you look at the 20,000-plus genes in each human and the interplay of the 140,000-plus toxins in the environment, spread among different genders, age groups, and their resiliency to other factors such as stress, the variables are too great for any reliable predictability.

Age

Age is yet an additional consideration when it comes to autoimmune diseases. Any of the various factors like gender, genetics, and the environment can have a different impact at different points in your life. The elderly may be more susceptible to environmental factors, either due to greater immune system dysregulation or greater accumulated exposures over time to environmental toxins. The effect of estrogen on women lessens as they age, which is represented by the fact that more women under the age of sixty-five are affected than those over. Certain exposures to triggering substances can have a greater impact at younger, rather than older ages.

What to Expect with a Diagnosis

Autoimmune conditions are not always easy to identify. Symptoms are not always unique to autoimmune conditions and may look like something else, or be so vague as to look like nothing else. This can often lead to patients being told that the condition is all in their heads. Looking for someone who specializes in autoimmune diseases can be very helpful. Be persistent and don't be afraid to seek a second or even third opinion.

Blood tests will typically look for the antibodies produced by the body's B cells. Certain blood markers can also show increased levels of inflammation that may affect organs like the liver or kidneys. Other diagnostic tools like x-rays, CT scans, and MRIs can be very useful, depending on the condition present.

ESSENTIAL

Misdiagnosis is a common problem in the medical field. It is more common than medication and surgical site errors. Millions of people are misdiagnosed each year. Misdiagnosis can also be a missed diagnosis. If symptoms continue, make sure that you consult another doctor for a second opinion.

It helps to be the most knowledgeable person about you in the room when you go to see a doctor. That means that you can clearly describe what makes your symptoms worse or better, how long you've had them, family history, etc. Know your own health history and bring along any past test results that you can. The complexity of autoimmune conditions requires as many pieces to the puzzle as possible. The doctor is solving a riddle and you and your observations can be the most important keys to solving it. Advocate for yourself, and if you aren't able to be your own advocate, have someone else do it on your behalf. The human body continues to be one of the biggest mysteries of life. Be a patient patient and know that you can always continue looking elsewhere for the answers you seek.

Medical Approach

From the medical perspective, most autoimmune conditions are viewed as lifelong conditions. Typically, anyone who is diagnosed with an autoimmune condition and follows the medical model of healthcare can expect to be treating it for the rest of her life.

Within the medical model, only the symptoms of autoimmune conditions can be addressed. The disease itself is viewed as too complicated in causation to treat successfully. Many approaches seek to suppress immune system function, which can leave the patient more vulnerable to infections. Some conditions may require blood transfusions or therapy to maintain mobility.

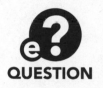

QUESTION

Has science discovered any ways to reverse autoimmune conditions? Scientists are continually working on discovering how autoimmunity begins in order to find ways to stop it. NAD+, a molecule that naturally exists in all living tissues, has the potential to reverse and protect against autoimmune diseases. Research in this area is new and NAD+ has yet to prove itself in clinical trials, but scientists are very hopeful.

Advancements in the field of medicine, however, may change this as newer technologies emerge. Scientists are hopeful about new therapies, but none have yet been shown to create substantial change. Researchers keep pushing ahead, as they realize that progress against any one condition is likely to be progress against all of them.

Holistic Approach

The holistic approach considers every aspect of the person and is centered on treating the person, not the disease. It considers as much as possible the totality, or whole person, and how everything interacts to produce health or disease. A holistic practitioner will consider everything a medical doctor considers and then also look at your lifestyle, stress levels, diet, nutrition, exercise, rest, and exposures to heavy metals and chemicals.

Diets

Diets should be primarily based on whole foods that are low- or noninflammatory in nature. This can vary from person to person according to the tissues involved, reactivity, and other components of their condition. What may be good for the majority of people may not work for a few people.

ALERT

The best diet will be the one that reduces or eliminates an overactive immune response. Each person's diet may need some fine-tuning in order to determine what works and what doesn't work. Use an autoimmune diet as the basis for controlling autoimmunity and then modify it according to your body's needs.

Most processed foods contain many ingredients that promote inflammation via various pathways in the body. Common allergens such as wheat, soy, nuts, dairy, and shellfish will create or add to autoimmune responses. Keep a list of foods that don't work for you. While some people may consider restrictive diets as too much of an inconvenience for their lifestyles, the alternatives of an unchecked progressive disease are less appealing.

Nutrition

Nutrition can sometimes be used as an intervention in the medical setting, but it tends to be more common with holistic practitioners. A holistic practitioner may recommend vitamins, herbs, minerals, and even homeopathy to address restoring health.

Detoxification

Detoxification is often recommended as a way to address the accumulation and effect of toxins in the body as a result of both internal and external pathways. Saunas have been shown to detoxify the body of heavy metals and many chemical compounds. Saunas have a long history of safe and proven benefits.

Stress

Stress is often a major factor in all conditions, but it is seldom addressed by mainstream medicine. This can also vary from person to person, as how you respond to any situation depends on a host of factors and personal history. Meditation, prayer, and yoga have been shown to lessen the effects of stress on a daily basis.

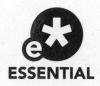

ESSENTIAL

Fortunately, stress can be addressed in a number of ways. A big key is to go slow and not rush or demand that your body responds faster than it is capable of. This only creates more stress and can delay, or even worsen, the healing process.

A holistic practitioner may make recommendations based on research or clinical evidence about certain techniques that have been shown to alleviate or diminish the effects of stress. These can include somatic therapy, EMDR, trauma release exercises (TRE), and the traditional cognitive (talk) therapies. Advancements in this area recognize that the body's response to past traumas and stress can play a much bigger role than previously thought.

The complexity of autoimmune conditions requires a broad view and consideration of everything taking place. Each of those can be a factor in restoring health. Having bias against any one or more areas can miss important information that needs to be considered.

CHAPTER 2

The Enemy Within

When we talk about autoimmune (AI) conditions, we focus on the body's immune responses and what causes the body to attack itself. An autoimmune attack is commonly believed to be the body's inability to recognize its own tissues and cells as separate from something else that's not normally found within the body. An AI attack can also be due to either the body missing some essential elements that help provide balanced responses or a loss of regulation of the immune system, leading to exaggerated responses. In short, the "enemy" within may be something foreign, or it may just be a sign of an imbalance that needs to be addressed.

Distinguishing the Body's Cells: Self versus Non-Self

The first tissues of the body are derived from the embryonic cells of a developing baby. These cells give rise to all the other cells and tissues that will make up the body and, in the process, establish what is a normal part of the body—the self—and what is not a normal part of the body—the non-self. The ability to recognize self versus non-self is considered to be at the heart of most autoimmune conditions. Like one big family, the system recognizes who is a part of the family and who isn't.

Self

The self, or human body, is an immensely complex organism that interacts and intersects through a vast network of checks and balances. Like a giant spider web, every cell, tissue, organ, and system is connected via a multitude of pathways. Anything that stimulates one part of this system is registered by every other part of the system. Each system of the self plays a vital role in creating a peaceful coexistence with every other part of the self.

ESSENTIAL

The complexity of the human body is thought by some to be finite given that it contains only so many cells, tissues, etc. Others view its complexity as infinite because it is engaged in a constantly evolving process that navigates the infinite complexity of the building blocks of life. However one views it, our understanding of it is extremely limited.

Within the self, the immune system is in charge of maintaining law and order. It helps ensure that we can go about our daily routines and operations without interference from outsiders. Armed with a wide variety of tools, it is prepared to respond to and meet any threat that should appear from an outside, or non-self, source. In order to do this, it has to be able to recognize not only self from non-self, but also human self from non-human self.

Human Self
Man doesn't typically consider himself to be anything other than human: flesh and blood, brain, liver, kidneys, stomach, and other organs, and all the

cells that make up each and every one of these. Each of them is a by-product of the master blueprint contained within the genetics of the first embryonic cells that formed us after conception. One grows out of the other until the human form takes shape and matures from there on. The thought of being a composite, or chimera, of different species is not usually a part of most people's viewpoint.

FACT

The chimera is a monstrous beast from Greek mythology. It is typically shown to have the head and body of a lion and a serpent tail, with the head of a goat arising from its back. The sphinx is one of the best known examples of a chimera.

Through observation and reflection, early man defined himself primarily by what was visible only to the eyes. Everything else was inconsequential. The man in the mirror, however, turned out to be a façade to an even more amazing and complex shadow in and around him. Instead of being a pureblood, man is a hybrid. The human self has a shadow side, the non-human self.

Nonhuman Self

The nonhuman self consists of all the microbes that are found on and in the body. There are over 100 trillion of them and they outnumber human cells by a factor of at least 10 to 1. Their genetics are more complex than human cells and outnumber man's genes by a factor of 360 to 1. With such an impressive resume, some scientists are stating that man is more microbe than he is human, while others call him a super-organism.

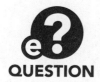

QUESTION

If antibiotics kill bacteria and they are essential for life, am I harming myself by taking them?
The use of any medication is considered in terms of a risk-to-benefit ratio. The short-term effect of antibiotics may be life-saving, but the long-term effect could be life-threatening. Always make sure the use of antibiotics is necessary, and never use them when it is not. Antibiotic resistance is the third leading threat to humanity.

These microbes play a vital role in the health of humans, and it can be argued that humans wouldn't exist without them, while they are not dependent on humans to exist. They have even been shown to ensure a full pregnancy, without which man would not exist. They inhabit the human body from birth and are with us throughout life and long afterward.

The immune system matures and develops under the influences of these microbes. They help create and develop tolerance within the immune system. In some autoimmune diseases, it is the loss of tolerance that can create the autoimmune response and subsequent damage that follows. Early theories stated that the immune system tolerates the presence of these microbes within the human body, but it is beginning to look like this relationship is much more complex and sophisticated than this simplistic viewpoint. It is beginning to look like man and microbe are simply two sides of the same coin. If you can't see both sides of the coin, one could make the mistake of thinking that the side being viewed is the only side, as was the case with early medicine.

Non-Self

Non-self can be anything that is not normally found in or on the body in the purest sense. It was originally believed to be anything that was not a human cell or fluid, but now we have developed a broader appreciation of what constitutes "man." If you consider the "good" microbes to be the ones that benefit man and thus are a part of the self, then the "bad" microbes are the ones that would harm the self or any of its components, and would be considered as non-self. In reality, this is another oversimplification, as the overall balance of the internal ecosystem that plays host to these 100 trillion microbes is a more important consideration than any one microbe alone.

ESSENTIAL

The human gut is considered "the densest ecosystem known in nature" by microbiologist Jeffrey Gordon. Certain bacteria have been associated with obesity, diabetes, and other conditions and functions, but these associations can shift as soon as the ecosystem within shifts. The sum effect can be more powerful than the individual effects.

Beyond microbes, non-self can also be the chemicals and heavy metals that find their way into the body and often create havoc for the body's tissues and cells. These substances can create an overwhelming burden on the body that can take time to resolve. Their presence is likely to cause a dysregulation of the immune system that leads to excessive responses and tissue damage.

In terms of the immune system, non-self elicits very powerful and rapid immune responses so as to maintain the overall balance and homeostasis of the body. When the response is excessive or dysregulated, autoimmunity results. In figuring out the best approach to resolving autoimmune conditions, it can be helpful to understand which part of the immune system is contributing to or causing the autoimmune reaction.

The Immune System's Toolbox

The immune system's toolbox is like an orchestra composed of many instruments with each one playing a thousand notes, all synchronized perfectly to create a harmonious movement. The complexity of the immune system is something that cannot be addressed in its entirety here, but a brief introduction to some of the components that play a role in inflammation, and therefore autoimmune diseases, can help create a clearer understanding of what takes place.

ALERT

Understanding how the immune system functions can help you make better choices about your lifestyle. Knowledge can be a tremendous tool for living a long, healthy life. Take time to learn more about the body so that you can make better decisions that empower and sustain your health. Complex knowledge requires baby steps in the beginning.

The first immune cells are unsophisticated, simple, naive cells that give rise to more sophisticated cells designed to produce a specific effect in an orchestrated immune response. This process of differentiation and maturation gives rise to the two arms of the immune system known as the innate and adaptive immune responses. Together, these two responses create immunity in the body. Although historically the adaptive response was considered the key player in autoimmunity, the innate response has now also been shown to play a vital role. These two arms of the immune system employ a host of mediators that help fine-tune the specific responses of each of the cells.

The Innate/Nonspecific Response

The innate, or nonspecific, response of the immune system is a very rapid response that does not create long-lasting protection. It is a spontaneous reaction by the immune system designed to eliminate any foreign substance that shouldn't be in the body. The innate cells include macrophages, neutrophils, dendritic cells, and the appropriately named natural killer (NK) cells, among others. Once the innate cells have done as much as possible to capture and render an intruder harmless, they then present samples of their victim's remains to the adaptive immune cells. These remnants are called antigens and help develop the adaptive immune response that follows.

Macrophage

Macrophages, from the Greek words meaning "big eater," are present in all tissues of the body. They roam around looking for foreign substances to eat, or engulf, a process called phagocytosis. They play a role in removing dead tissues and cells, orchestrating immune cell responses, repairing wounds, and maintaining homeostasis. They can be either inflammatory (M1 macrophages) or anti-inflammatory (M2 macrophages) in their response, depending on the environment they find themselves in and the signals they receive.

The spleen is a large reservoir for the body's macrophages. In addition to their immune system roles, macrophages that are stored in the spleen have been found to play a role in the repair of heart tissues after a heart attack. The spleen's other roles include filtering blood, weeding out parasites and old cells, and recycling iron.

Macrophages have different forms and functions as well as names, depending on the tissues in which they exist. They are known as Kupffer and stellate cells in the liver, microglia in the brain, Langerhans in the skin, and so on. Macrophages are a vital part of the immune system response, powerhouses capable of devouring most anything in their path. The macrophage isn't without its Achilles' heel, however, as some pathogens are able to exploit the macrophage for their own growth and development. *Candida albicans* is a good example of a pathogen that can manipulate the macrophage at will.

Neutrophil

Neutrophils are the most abundant white blood cells present in humans. They reside predominantly in the blood stream until they are recruited via special proteins called chemokines to enter the tissues and assist in elimination of pathogens.

They are strong drivers of inflammation and can be responsible for tissue damage if left unchecked. Neutrophils are true killing machines that utilize a wide variety of tools to accomplish their tasks. Like the macrophages, they can engulf and neutralize substances. When this is not possible, they can secrete enzymes, peptides, reactive oxygen species, and even their own DNA into surrounding fluids and tissues. Neutrophil extracellular traps (NETs) are composed of secreted neutrophil DNA that entraps pathogens in a web to immobilize them for other immune cells to finish off.

Dendritic Cells

Dendritic cells (DCs) engulf substances and then present their antigen remnants to other cells of the adaptive immune system. In this role, like macrophages, they are called antigen-presenting cells (APCs), and act as a messenger between the two sides of the immune response.

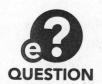

QUESTION

Where do dendritic cells come from?
Dendritic cells, like all other white blood cells, come from the bone marrow. Most are formed in the red marrow of bones while some are formed in the yellow marrow. Yellow marrow is higher in fat and tends to replace red marrow as we age.

When not acting as a messenger they can be found directing other immune responses like the general of an army. While there is still much to be learned about these immune cells, research implicates them in the development of most autoimmune conditions.

Natural Killer Cells

The appropriately named natural killer (NK) cells are specialized immune cells that target cancer cells and cells infected with viruses. They can be found interacting with macrophages, DCs, and T cells to accomplish this task and others. Like other immune cells, they can increase or decrease immune system responses, especially those involving inflammation. NK cells are believed to play a role in causing, maintaining, or increasing autoimmune diseases. The exact role is not yet known, but some studies show that it is a deficiency of NK cells that may be associated with the excessive responses found in autoimmunity.

Other Innate Cells

Other innate immune cells include mast cells, eosinophils, basophils, and even the cells of the body's natural barriers in the skin, urinary, respiratory, and intestinal tracts. Apart from acting as natural barriers, much of what these cells do, when not engulfing foreign intruders, has been associated with conditions like allergies and asthma through their pro-inflammatory responses. Though small in number, their influence can be mighty, as anyone with asthma and seasonal allergies can attest to. Depending on the environment and the signals they receive, they can play a role in both innate and adaptive immunity.

The Adaptive/Specific Response

The adaptive response is wired to produce a long-lasting memory of previous infections. While initially slower than the innate response, once memory has been developed, it allows for a fast and specifically targeted response to any repeat exposures to previously encountered infectious agents, chemicals, or other non-self substances.

ESSENTIAL

The specific, or adaptive, immune response is not yet present when babies are born. This response develops over time and is one reason that vaccines aren't believed to be as effective in newborns as they are in adults.

It is the adaptive response and its production of antibodies that is most commonly associated with autoimmunity. The commonly held belief is that the body misidentifies its own tissue as a foreign substance or antigen and then produces antibodies to the cells and tissues of the body. This point of view is unlikely to be sustained, as it views the body as not knowing what it is doing (a common perspective in medicine when faced with a lack of understanding and knowledge about what's taking place in the body). It is more likely that something else is taking place that science has yet to decipher and the immune system is simply doing what it is designed to do, albeit under conditions that render it incapable of functioning in a regulated way.

T Cells

T cells are white blood cells that are named after the thymus gland where they mature after being birthed in the bone marrow. There are several types of T cells, also known as T helper (Th) cells. Some of the main ones frequently discussed include Th1, Th2, Th17, and Tregs.

FACT

T cells are produced in the bone marrow and travel to the thymus gland, where most of them mature. A small amount of T cells mature in the tonsils. The thymus gland shrinks during the aging process, which can lead to immune system dysregulation and autoimmune disease.

Th1 and Th17 are typically considered to be very pro-inflammatory in their function, whereas Th2 and Tregs are more likely to help modulate or decrease inflammatory responses. Of course, it's never just one way in the body and all of these cells, under the right conditions, may switch their roles.

Given such diversity, it is no wonder that science is still unable to produce consistent results with any reliability.

B Cells

The B cells are primarily involved in the production of antibodies, except when they're not. B cells can also fill in as antigen-presenting cells (APCs) when needed. Once the B cell has become activated, it can turn into either a plasma cell or a memory cell. The plasma cells are efficient at producing large amounts of antibodies, while the memory cells are conditioned to respond to specific antigens/intruders for a long time. These two cells can play a role in lifelong immunity and health or lifelong autoimmunity and disease.

Immune Cell Mediators

Chemokines, interleukins, complement proteins, antibodies, etc., make up the list of mediators, or cytokines, that form a cascade of responses from immune cells throughout the body, or locally within specific tissues. The list of immune cell mediators is a work in progress. Science is continually discovering new mediators and the immune cells that produce them. In keeping with much of the common battle terminology used when speaking about the immune system, immune cells are the guns and the mediators are the bullets.

QUESTION

Are there any drugs to counteract cytokines?
Yes, cytokines tend to be a primary target for reducing inflammation. One problem that arises from their use is that even cytokines that are very pro-inflammatory will also play an anti-inflammatory role and often help maintain homeostasis of the immune system. Targeting cytokines often creates other problems.

In general, someone who is ill produces more cytokines more frequently and is likely to be more symptomatic. Certain mediators are pro-inflammatory, while others are anti-inflammatory. In a balanced response, the pro-inflammatory response will be regulated and buffered by the anti-inflammatory response. In immune system dysregulation, inflammation will be unchecked, prolonged, and more likely to create disease.

Interleukins

Interleukins are cytokines that play a large role in the function of the immune system, especially as communicators between white blood cells, also known as leukocytes. As many of them activate certain white blood cells, they play a role in the inflammatory process. IL-1, IL-6, and IL-17 are especially known for their ability to stimulate inflammation in the body. IL-10 on the other hand is anti-inflammatory by its ability to inhibit the production of many cytokines.

Chemokines

Chemokines are signaling proteins that help direct cells where to go. As far as the immune system is concerned, they act as guide dogs that enable white blood cells to home in on infected tissues. This migration toward a site is called chemotaxis. Chemokines can recruit specific immune cells needed to handle specific infections, as is the case with neutrophils being recruited to eliminate a candida infection. In response, candida has developed the ability to block the release of chemokines in order to avoid having to deal with neutrophils.

TNF-alpha

TNF-alpha is a powerful cytokine and a strong driver of inflammation and tissue destruction in the body. Like everything else, it is not completely understood yet, but it has a variety of functions. It can destroy tumor cells and induce fevers or even cause cell death. It is commonly involved in runaway bloodstream infections called sepsis and the wasting away of the body as seen in AIDS and cancers.

Complement Proteins

Complement proteins are a group of small proteins that are typically produced by the liver and function as a part of both the innate and adaptive immune responses. They help amplify immune responses and function via three known pathways that determine their role in an immune response.

ESSENTIAL

Complement proteins can make a bad situation worse by amplifying inflammation levels. This happens in sepsis when infections set up in the bloodstream. The immune response amplified by complement proteins can lead to death. In this case, the immune response can be more dangerous than the infection.

Complement proteins are believed to play a role in many autoimmune diseases. It is a tightly regulated systemic network that can create a lot of tissue damage in autoimmune diseases.

Antibodies

Antibodies are proteins produced in response to antigens. As such they help direct specific responses that target future exposures to the same antigens. When antibodies are developed against human tissues, autoimmunity develops. Antibodies, or immunoglobulins (Ig), are typically secreted by the large plasma cells. There are five main types of antibodies:

1. IgM
2. IgG
3. IgA
4. IgD
5. IgE

IgM is associated with early infection responses, while IgG develops later. A positive finding of IgM on a blood test can indicate that someone has a current infection, while IgG indicates a previous infection. IgA indicates that cells of the mucus system are involved and is generally found with intestinal, respiratory, and urinary tract infections. IgE is commonly found with allergic reactions and also parasites, while IgD is not usually considered, as it relates to B cells that have yet to be activated.

Elevated levels of Igs on blood tests generally indicate some type of disease or infectious process. If an infection has been around for a long time, however, the immune response becomes exhausted and can alter the findings on blood tests.

Many doctors only look for elevated levels of Igs on blood tests and will miss out on the significance of suppressed or, occasionally, normal levels. A blood test is only a snapshot in time and should be referenced against previous or later blood tests for a more accurate picture.

Friend or Foe? Immune System Responses

The immune system plays a vital role in protecting you from external and internal threats, as it differentiates friend from foe. It must have the ability to defend the body against massive attacks, and at the same time be able to hunt down the smallest cell or substance that doesn't belong. At all times, it must be able to regulate its own activity and modify its responses so that no collateral damage is done to friendly tissues or even to itself. It must develop a tolerance to the 100 trillion microbial cells that are a part of the human body and be able to recognize self from non-self. When these abilities break down, autoimmunity can develop.

Molecular Mimicry

The prevailing opinion on autoimmunity that you're likely to hear from your doctor is that the body mistakes its own tissues as being the cause of an imbalance and thereafter attacks that tissue, resulting in a disease or condition. This is known as molecular mimicry. The body tissue being attacked is similar to, or mimicking, part of a virus, bacteria, or other pathogen, and the body can't tell the difference.

Molecular mimicry has been a popular theory in autoimmune diseases for over 30 years and is still considered the primary hypothesis as to how autoimmune disease develops. Rheumatic fever is the classic model for molecular mimicry as it typically develops after a respiratory infection with streptococcus bacteria that cross-react with cardiac tissues.

Another way that this can happen is that during an infection of some tissue of the body, the white blood cells identify both the infectious pathogen and the body's tissue together and so create antibodies to both. From that point on, it will attack either one should they reappear, and in the case of a tissue in the body, it's always present and so lifelong autoimmunity develops.

One challenge to this theory is that the body has always known the tissue as self and so therefore it should continue to recognize it as self and not attack it.

Aging and Senescence

Senescence of the immune system is a process of deterioration that occurs with aging. The immune system requires tight regulation. Deterioration of any one part or several parts, as happens with aging, can lead to a loss of the regulation needed to maintain balance and tolerance. Without homeostasis the system begins to collapse upon itself.

Chronic low-grade inflammation is common in the elderly. Pro-inflammatory levels of IL-6 and TNF-alpha are increased. Antibody production by B cells often decreases. The aging body can struggle to create balance in the immune system. This can also be due to decreased absorption of nutrients needed to sustain proper immune system function.

Stress

Stress can cause dysregulation of the immune system. Stress and trauma can increase cortisol and other stress-related hormone levels in the body, which in turn suppress and dysregulate immune system function via altered cytokine production. Stress therapies have been shown to improve autoimmune conditions. Autoimmune conditions themselves create stress, which then adds to the disease process.

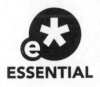

ESSENTIAL

Stress is often associated with playing a role in almost all diseases, either as a causative or an exacerbating agent. Some sources state that 80–90 percent of all diseases are caused by stress. Heart disease is commonly associated with the effects of stress on the body.

Carnegie Mellon University researcher Sheldon Cohen states: "When under stress, cells of the immune system are unable to respond to hormonal control, and consequently, produce levels of inflammation that promote disease." Stress and trauma can cause ongoing, lifelong imbalances that can be reflected in an autoimmune disease. That stress promotes autoimmune disease is generally accepted, but how that happens is still not clear.

Medication

Many medications are linked to autoimmune diseases. Antibiotics are linked to several autoimmune diseases due to their effect on the 100 trillion bacteria of the intestinal tract, wherein lies approximately 70 percent of the body's immune system. Chemotherapy can often cause autoimmune conditions. Drugs that seek to suppress certain immune responses can cause autoimmune disease. Statin drugs for high cholesterol have been linked to autoimmune disease. With an average of over 398 side effects per medication, medications can be a leading cause of autoimmune disease.

Nutrient Deficiency

Nutritional imbalances are another cause of autoimmune diseases. Vitamins, minerals, proteins, and fats can all affect immune system homeostasis. Antioxidant minerals and vitamins can help repair autoimmune damage and modulate immune system function. Vitamins A, C, D, and E play a role in both innate and adaptive immunity.

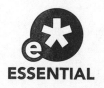

ESSENTIAL

Vitamin D is one of the most important vitamins when it comes to inflammation and autoimmunity. It is considered the anti-autoimmune vitamin. Making sure to get plenty of exposure to sunshine on a daily basis is an excellent way to prevent vitamin D deficiency.

Researchers at St. Thomas's Hospital in London have stated, "Nutrition and nutritional status can have profound effects on immune functions, resistance to infection and autoimmunity in man and other animals. Nutrients enhance or depress immune function depending on the nutrient and level of its intake."

Toxic Burden

The body accumulates toxins quite easily over a lifetime from ongoing daily exposures. Chemicals and heavy metals have both been associated with increased levels of autoimmunity via their effects on both innate and adaptive immunity. Mercury, cadmium, aluminum, and lead have been linked with autoimmune diseases. Chemicals in excess of 140,000 are added to the environment each year with very little research into their effects on immunity and other areas of health. A few like dioxins, carbon monoxide, polychlorinated biphenyls (PCBs), polycyclic aromatic hydrocarbons (PAHs), and many others are known to alter immune responses.

Food-related toxins and compounds are also linked to autoimmunity. Gluten and genetically modified organisms can influence immunity and inflammation. Sugar is a strong promoter of inflammation in the body.

Worm Food: Helminthic Therapy Research

A large area of current scientific interest is the effects of microbes on health and immunity. Oversterilization of our environment has altered the normal habitat in which man has coexisted with microbes for millions of years. Lifestyle changes in industrialized countries and the constant use of antimicrobials and disinfectants, along with decreased exposure to infectious agents, has resulted in increases in autoimmune and allergic diseases. This orientation toward excessive cleanliness and its effect on health is called the hygiene hypothesis, or "old friends" theory.

Studies have shown that the incidence of autoimmune allergic diseases is higher in countries with more sanitation, not less. Autoimmune conditions like type 1 diabetes, atopic dermatitis, multiple sclerosis, irritable bowel syndrome, Crohn's, and others, have a greater association with more hygienic environments. Making matters worse, medicine has not been able to find an answer to the rising toll of these diseases on society.

Studies have shown that where the exposure to parasites is higher, the occurrence of autoimmune diseases is lower. This appears to be particularly true of helminth parasites, a type of parasite that is known to live in the intestinal tract of humans without causing any disease or sickness.

I thought worms were the cause of diseases worldwide. How are helminth worms any safer?
Helminth and certain other types of worms are known to down-regulate and block inflammation and autoimmune disease in the body much in the same way as some of the body's interleukins. It is reasoned that helminths have been a part of the human digestive tract for thousands of years, helping keep humans healthy, as opposed to other types of worms that can be problematic.

Researchers around the globe have found that giving helminths to sick individuals can induce a high cure rate. At the University of Iowa, Dr. Joel Weinstock found that giving test subjects with Crohn's disease a weekly drink containing thousands of parasite eggs could induce an almost 75 percent cure rate. Elsewhere, similar studies at Harvard, University of California San Francisco, Trinity College Dublin, Glasgow and Edinburgh Universities, and others found high success rates with autoimmune conditions such as multiple sclerosis, autism, celiac, allergies, type 1 diabetes, and dermatitis.

The success of helminthic therapy has generated the establishment of support groups on the Internet at such sites as Facebook and Yahoo!, where members share their stories and successes on a daily basis.

In one sense, autoimmunity may simply be an indication that humans are no longer in sync with their environment. In the past, humans feared their environment and sought to separate themselves from it as much as possible, fearing that bacteria, parasites, and other organisms could only cause illness. Now, that trend is reversing itself as many people are getting back to healthier choices that include interacting more with nature and all the microbes that are a part of that natural environment. Getting dirty is being appreciated in new ways.

CHAPTER 3

The Environmental Impact

A common definition for the environment is "the sum total of all surroundings of a living organism, including natural forces and other living things, which provide conditions for development and growth, as well as danger and damage." Although the link between man and his environment is just beginning to be uncovered, the early results have not been favorable. The give-and-take scenario is being shown to have a tremendous effect on human health and disease. With the rates of autoimmune diseases continuing to increase yearly, it is imperative that we have a better understanding of what is taking place.

Is It Your Environment or Your Genetics?

Which came first, the chicken or the egg? The chicken or the egg question is one that reveals the complexity and interwoven nature of life. Where does one begin and the other one end? This dilemma is also found with humans and our environment. As we are a part of the environment, where do you draw the line between the two?

The old philosophy was that man was separate from his environment and evolved above it, or was given dominion over it, to do with as he pleased without ever needing to consider the consequence of his actions. We have now seen that this is not the case, as it appears that everything that we do impacts nature and nature in return impacts us.

The chain of life on this planet is interconnected down to the smallest molecule and atom. Rachel Carson's 1962 groundbreaking book *Silent Spring* awakened the collective consciousness of man to the effects of poisoning the planet and everything that lives upon it. No longer could we continue as unwitting participants in the destruction of the circle of life on this planet. As science continued to advance in this area, we became aware that we were a part of this circle of life, and our reckless concern for nature was proving to be our downfall as well.

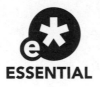

ESSENTIAL

Rachel Carson is credited with starting the environmental movement with the publication of her book *Silent Spring*. The book details the effects of DDT and several other common toxins of the day that were wreaking havoc on nature and animals. It was immediately a bestseller that was supported by then-president John F. Kennedy.

With the ongoing evolution of all fields of science, we have more clearly etched out a basic understanding of the impact of the chemicals and toxins that are released into the environment on a daily, monthly, and yearly basis. Upon this sketchy framework, we are discovering more and more about our impact on the environment, and therefore ultimately upon us as well. Science is working to differentiate this environmental impact on man against a background of genetic influence. Where autoimmunity is concerned, is it the environment or genetics?

Genetics

It was a long-held belief that one day we would learn the makeup of the human genetic tree, or genome, and have all the answers to disease and health. That day has come and gone and we are no closer to having all our questions answered, which only leaves us with even more questions. Advancements in science have allowed us to see deeper into the structure and function of the cells and the DNA strands of our genetics. We know even more about the building blocks of life than we've ever known. We have a bigger picture of the smaller pieces, but still find ourselves lacking in our understanding, which leaves a lot open to observation and interpretation.

FACT

The Human Genome Project was started in 1984 and involved an international group of scientists from twenty universities. Completed in 2003, it mapped out about 20,000 human genes, much less than the 100,000-plus genes that it was expected to find.

Genetic clues to autoimmune disease continue to reveal themselves. Variations in certain genes have been associated with certain autoimmune conditions. Multiple genes combined together have been associated with contributing to a greater "risk" of getting a condition, while individually these genes seem to have very little effect. Among multiple autoimmune conditions there are some common genes that frequently occur among people of the same race, sex, or geography. The prevalence of autoimmune diseases in certain families is another indication of a genetic effect handed down from one generation to another. The catalog of genes and autoimmunity is still being assembled, gene by gene. How close or far away we are from having all the answers is unknown.

Environment

When speaking about the environment versus genetics, a scientist is really looking at the impact of the environment on genetics, an epigenetic effect. What is the epigenetic effect? Professor Marcus Pembrey put forth the best definition of epigenetics: "It is a change in our genetic activity without changing our genetic code." The genes are there, but they can be turned on and off, amplified or silenced.

Like a tree or bush, our genetics are always being pruned, one way or another, toward health or disease. The effect of an outer influence on how our genes behave can be handed down from generation to generation, the same as genetics themselves. Each new generation will be faced with environmental factors that can affect both their genes and the factors that previously affected their parents' genes.

QUESTION

If someone in my family has an autoimmune condition, will I get it also? Although family members are more likely to have autoimmune conditions if someone else in their family has one, it's not so common that you should be afraid of it happening. Epigenetics have demonstrated this in studies of twins that have identical traits, but don't develop the same conditions, if any. The epigenetic effect of one's lifestyle may turn on or off certain genes.

As Italian researchers recently stated, "Many autoimmune diseases are brought out by other risk factors, some of which are preventable. The most common preventable aggravators of autoimmune diseases include infections, smoking, and heavy alcohol consumption." Another study found that a high-salt diet can drive the production of highly inflammable immune cells like Th17, GM-CSF, and TNF-alpha. Other studies continue to link a wide variety of factors with autoimmune diseases. Mood disorders later on in life were linked to infections and autoimmune conditions during childhood.

Chemicals and heavy metals, like mercury, also exert their epigenetic effect, as does stress or trauma. The average individual is swimming in a sea of epigenetic factors throughout every minute of his life. In its broadest sense, everything in life has the potential to affect you in one way or another.

Fortunately, it's not all bad. Just as toxins and stress can exert a negative effect on genetics, so too can antioxidants, fruit, veggies, vitamins, and minerals exert a positive influence. The average human is engaged in a daily seesaw battle back and forth on the playground of genetics.

FACT

The effects of epigenetics can often be found at the very beginning of life, while the child is still developing within the mother's womb. Changes at this stage of life have been linked to transgenerational changes that may not show up until the child grows up and has her own children.

Toxins Are Passed from Mother to Child

In the past, every doctor was taught that the mother's womb is a virtually pristine environment that protects the developing baby from toxins that the mom may be exposed to or that are already embedded in the tissues of the mother's body. This protection is accomplished by the barrier of the umbilical cord that ferries nutrients and other necessary building blocks of life to the baby. Although the essential ingredients may pass, nothing else was ever supposed to breach this barrier.

All of that changed in 2004 when a study from the Environmental Working Group (EWG) revealed that this pristine lifeline had been hijacked by industrial wastes, pollutants, and toxins. Of the 400 or so chemicals tested for, an average of 200 chemicals per baby was discovered in the umbilical cord blood of the babies at birth. A total of 287 chemicals out of 417 were found in these babies, representing a toxic load of over 68 percent. How many of the hundreds of thousands of chemicals would have been found if they had all been tested for?

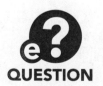

QUESTION

Do toxins affect babies differently than adults?
For most of the history of medicine, science viewed a baby's body as just a smaller version of an adult body. This was found not to be true, as there are many differences. A baby's body is less able to respond to and handle toxins the way an adult can. With less body mass toxins can have a more damaging effect on a baby's tissues and the genetics that affect later generations.

Environmental toxins have reached what was considered the last pristine environment on the planet. Babies are being born pre-polluted, never having had the opportunity to know what a world without toxins is like.

The baby's toxic journey starts at the moment of conception. As the new cells divide and double, the baby's body emerges and takes its form. The cells of a baby are developing at a rapid pace and the effects of toxins at this point can be much greater during this rapid growth phase than later on when everything is set and the body's defenses are in place. Considering this, one can look at the effects of some of the toxins discovered in the EWG study with much greater appreciation, and perhaps fear.

Mercury

Mercury is one of the well-known environmental toxins that many people try to avoid. Long gone are the days when kids used to play with the mercury in thermometers. People are careful about how much and which fish they eat, as well as what type of fillings they allow dentists to use when putting in fillings for cavities.

ALERT

Dental fillings that contain mercury amalgam, the silver-colored fillings, are listed on government websites as releasing "low levels of mercury vapor that can be inhaled." Holistic healthcare practitioners recommend removing all mercury fillings and replacing them with composite materials that are hypoallergenic.

Mercury has long been known for its neurotoxicity and more recently, its ability to act as an immune system toxin has become better established. Occupational exposures have linked mercury with autoimmune lupus.

Animal studies have linked mercury to immune system dysfunction, autoimmune myocarditis, arthritis, and autoimmune thyroiditis. Whether mercury directly causes autoimmunity or indirectly through an increase in antibodies has not been clearly established. At some level however, it appears to be playing a role in increasing autoimmunity.

Polyaromatic Hydrocarbons

Polyaromatic hydrocarbons (PAHs), or polycyclic aromatic hydrocarbons, are environmental toxins that are known carcinogens and immunotoxins. They commonly occur as a by-product of burning coal, gasoline, wood, tobacco, and garbage. They can also be found in roofing tar, creosote, pesticides, and plastics. Like many other toxins, they are also linked to autoimmune thyroiditis.

FACT

Polyaromatic hydrocarbons (PAHs) are everywhere in the environment and very difficult to avoid. They have been linked to liver, lung, and skin damage leading to cancers. They can create a dysregulation of the immune system that can play a role in autoimmune conditions. Unconsciousness and convulsions are two other effects from prolonged exposure.

Absorption of PAHs can occur through the respiratory and GI tracts, and the skin. Immune system effects can include increases in inflammatory immune cells. PAHs are commonly found in water where their removal is difficult to achieve through conventional community water treatment facilities.

Per- and Polyfluorinated Compounds

Polyfluorinated chemicals (PFCs) are found in waterproofing and flame retardant materials used in clothing and furniture. Additional uses include nonstick cookware, electronics, textiles, food wraps, and construction materials. PFCs can last in the body for several years and have been linked to cancer, birth defects, autoimmunity, diabetes, neuropathy, and infertility. PFCs can last for decades in the environment and are a global problem, with at least 10,000 tons being produced every year.

Organochlorine Pesticides

Organochlorine pesticides (OCs) include the infamously banned toxin DDT, as well as chlordane, aldrin, dieldrin, heptachlor, lindane, and dioxins like TCDD that were used in Agent Orange during the Vietnam War. OCs are known to cause cancers, infertility, seizures, tremors, Parkinson's, and immune system abnormalities. Many of the organochlorine pesticides are no longer in use, although they still persist in the environment and continue to show up in testing of the body's fluids and tissues decades later.

ESSENTIAL

The organochlorine pesticide DDT is still being used in some countries. North Korea and India are two of the few remaining countries that permit its production and use. While use of this pesticide was banned worldwide, except in small quantities, several countries are now preparing to reintroduce its use once again.

Organochlorine pesticides have demonstrated high levels of estrogenic activity, which is known to drive cancers and autoimmunity.

Polychlorinated Naphthalenes

Polychlorinated naphthalenes (PCNs) are familiar to most people who have moth problems, as PCNs are found in mothproofing materials. Levels in the environment persist even though usage has been reduced greatly due to their toxic effects on humans. PCNs can still be found in wood preservatives and varnishes. Their toxicity is primarily associated with liver and kidney damage.

Polychlorinated Biphenyls

Polychlorinated biphenyls (PCBs) were banned in the United States many years ago but still persist in the environment in the air, water, and soils. PCBs were originally used in manufacturing electric and hydraulic equipment, pigments, dyes, oil-based paints, carbonless paper, adhesives and tapes. Items made with PCBs prior to the 1979 ban are still found in many buildings. Over 1.5 billion pounds are still a part of the environment. PCBs are associated with causing cancers, nervous system and reproductive disorders, and altered thyroid and immune system function.

Polybrominated Diphenyl Ethers

Polybrominated diphenyl ethers (PBDEs) have been used as flame retardants in furniture, television and computer casings, and textiles. Primary absorption appears to be from dietary sources and ingestion. PBDEs are known to affect the nervous and immune systems, causing alterations in immune cell signaling. They can trigger autoimmune thyroid disease due to the similarity of their structure with that of the thyroid hormone, thyroxine (T4).

These toxins are just a brief sampling of the 200 that were found in the EWG study, and an even more nominal example of the thousands, or even tens of thousands, that are likely to exist within pregnant mothers and, therefore, in their developing babies as well.

The Burden of Environmental Toxins

The burden of environmental toxins appears to be much larger than our ability to handle it. Millions of tons of chemicals persist in the environment many decades after they were banned in the United States and elsewhere. Hundreds of thousands of tons are being added to the environment every year, globally.

ALERT

Many people think that they are not being affected by the toxins in their environment, in spite of the overwhelming quantities that they are exposed to daily. It can take days, weeks, months, and years for symptoms to show up, often not until a lot of damage has been done. It's best to take a proactive role in creating optimal health.

Chemical Roulette

How, where, and when these chemical toxins will affect each person is unknown. It's a game of roulette in which everyone loses.

The Occupational Safety and Health Administration (OSHA) estimates that in the United States, "over 30 million workers are exposed to hazardous chemicals in their workplaces." Over 650,000 chemicals make up the list of toxins that threaten their health and livelihood. On an even larger scale, there are over 90 million registered organic and inorganic substances around the world. Every 3–4 seconds, another chemical is added to the list of millions of others on the American Chemical Society website. Together, these substances create a toxic stew that man now finds himself floating in.

Man is a sponge to his environment and the sum of these toxic substances has the potential to saturate all the tissues of the human body and lead to dysfunction and dysregulation of cells, tissues, organs, and systems, beyond the body's ability to cope and adapt. This inability to adapt is reflected in the ever-increasing number of people being saddled with autoimmune disease and illness.

Medicated Risk

When disease and illness are present in today's world, the most common choice is to take medications that only serve to address the symptoms and not the cause. The medications themselves are yet another source of toxicity, with each one having various side effects.

QUESTION

Are there medications that are safe to take with autoimmune conditions?
Every medication has its own set of risks. Medications that are anti-inflammatory in nature are designed to reduce autoimmune symptoms. All medications can also induce the very conditions that they are taken to treat. This is called the "paradoxical effect."

In 2012, researchers at Stanford University found an average of 329 new side effects per medication for every one of the 1,332 medications in their database. Prior to this, the average number of known side effects per drug was 69. Together, this means that the average number of side effects per drug is somewhere in the neighborhood of 398. That's a hard pill to swallow when the average human body is already loaded with toxins. As chemicals are mixed with more chemicals with no idea as to how they interact, the human chemistry experiment continues.

Processed Foods

Processed foods are a by-product of an industrialized society. As societies grew and became more complex, they needed foods that were more convenient and easier to prepare, with extended shelf lives for easy storage. To help accomplish this feat, processing methods required the addition of chemicals for various purposes. Over time, the list of chemicals being used in food processing has grown to over 10,000. From dyes, flavors, and preservatives, to even substitutes for the real food, today's processed foods have very little in common with the whole foods.

FACT

> The American refrigerator is the hallmark of America's processed food lifestyle. It is at least two to three times the size of its European counterpart and runs day and night. It is a long way from the iceboxes of the earlier part of the twentieth century and is symbolic of America's consumer-driven lifestyle.

Today, these chemical food additives and replacements have become associated with autoimmune conditions. Many of them are exactly the same as ones found in medications. Their main area of absorption is the intestinal tract. Some exert their influence on the intestinal barrier, leading to increased permeability and absorption of substances that should never cross this barrier into the bloodstream. Some are suspected of contributing to Crohn's and irritable bowel syndrome.

One of the best-known additives, refined salt, has been associated with increased levels of inflammation via its effect on the pro-inflammatory Th17 immune cells. Researchers at Yale University found that mice exposed to a diet high in refined salts were more likely to develop symptoms similar to multiple sclerosis in humans. Other common additives that many people find to be problematic include MSG, aspartame, saccharin, artificial coloring and preservatives, sodium benzoate and nitrate, and high-fructose corn syrup. Each of these additives has been found to contribute to and magnify levels of inflammation in the body that can add to already inflamed tissues and rapidly progressing disease processes.

MSG is a common additive found in many foods. It is believed to drive inflammation of the body that leads to liver damage, obesity, and diabetes. Many people are sensitive to MSG and avoid it when dining out. As it is pro-inflammatory, a good general rule to follow is to avoid it during times of sickness.

Outnumbered and overwhelmed, the immune system seems to act as though burning everything to the ground through increased levels of chronic inflammation is the only recourse left to it.

Unique Problems Humans Face

Today we are faced with navigating the maze of choices that presents itself to us on a daily basis. Where to live and work? What and how much to eat? How much time to spend exercising, sleeping, and resting? Each decision creates an impact that can advance or reverse the process of inflammation and autoimmune diseases in the body. In many ways, we are no longer matched to the environment that we have created for ourselves. There can be disadvantages in every situation that need to be considered.

Women and Toxins

Women seem to struggle more with autoimmune diseases than men do. Much of that is believed to be due to the effects of hormones and specifically those of estrogen. Estrogen has been shown to activate and enhance several autoimmune conditions.

Many chemicals mimic the effects of estrogen in the body. This is accomplished when certain molecules contained within the structure of chemicals bind to estrogen receptors on cells and stimulate the cells in the same way that estrogen would. Unlike naturally produced estrogen in the body, these chemical molecules often persist much longer in their effect and with greater magnitude.

This becomes particularly challenging for women, as many of the toxins in the environment possess estrogenic activity. These toxins will exert an influence upon the cells and tissues of the body in the exact same manner as estrogen. The FDA's Estrogenic Activity Database lists the estrogenic activity of thousands of chemicals.

By the time a woman reaches the age of sixty, her normal estrogen levels have decreased significantly and her incidence of autoimmune diseases declines as well. At the same time, a man's production of estrogen increases as he ages, creating greater risk factors for him in developing autoimmune conditions.

Location, Location, Location

Where you live should be a big consideration when it comes to any risk of autoimmune diseases. Urban centers are becoming notorious for the large amounts of toxins being released into the air, waterways, and soils. Study after study highlights the dangers of living in larger cities where traffic patterns exert tremendous pressures on the likelihood of contracting a disease as a result of air pollution.

Living closer to roads and highways has been associated with several diseases. Researchers from Canada found that living within 1,000 meters (3,280 feet) was linked to greater risks of bronchitis, asthma, and obstructive airway disease. Other studies have shown an increased risk of cardiovascular disease, cancers, and death. During rush-hour traffic, emergency room visits increase for people living within 300 meters of a major roadway. Other studies have shown that the small particulate matter that makes up air pollutants can increase inflammation and autoimmunity in conditions such as lupus and rheumatoid arthritis. Researchers from Canada found that air pollution can have a systemic effect on inflammation that even reaches as far as the bone marrow.

Communities that are surrounded by major industrial centers face additional risks. Living near gas production facilities or any number of other industries that routinely release toxins into the air and water compromises the quality of life, and can even shorten it. Sometimes living near such centers is not required, as wind and weather patterns can play a role in dispersing toxins over great distances to unsuspecting communities.

Cause and effect is a poor model for healthcare, as the effects of exposure to chemicals may not produce symptoms for a long time, up to years and decades. Inflammation commonly exists in the body at levels that are not registered consciously. Researchers from Germany and Switzerland found that air pollution from traffic and industrial sources can lead to asymptomatic increases in inflammation.

Antibiotics and the Gut

Most people in civilized societies have had multiple exposures to antibiotic medications, directly and indirectly. This can create lifelong alterations to the bacterial flora of the gut that lead to chronic inflammatory conditions. Chronic inflammation leads to a breakdown of the gut barriers that then allows substances to pass into the rest of the body via the circulation. This "leaky gut" condition has been associated with a multitude of autoimmune conditions.

Harvard researcher Sushrut Jangi, MD, states, "MS has more in common with inflammatory bowel disease, rheumatoid arthritis, lupus, and some of the other immune diseases than neurodegenerative diseases." In another study at Massachusetts General Hospital, in conjunction with the Broad Institute, researchers were able to identify specific bacteria involved with Crohn's disease. The researchers in this study questioned the practice of using antibiotics in the treatment of Crohn's: "We question this practice based on our observation that the microbial network appears [negatively disrupted] in the context of antibiotic exposure. Loss of protective microbes has the potential of triggering a proliferation of less beneficial taxa, exacerbating the inflammation."

A study from the University of British Columbia demonstrated that antibiotic use early in life can alter lifelong immunity. Another study on the early use of antibiotics showed that it can also predispose one to altered metabolism and obesity later in life. The gut contains approximately 70 percent of the body's immune system. The microbiome plays a big role in the health of this system and therefore the health of the body. Altering the bacterial flora will have lifelong effects and can impact autoimmunity. Careful consideration must be exercised when weighing the pros and cons of their use.

CHAPTER 4

A Difficult Diagnosis

The process of identifying any disease or condition is a difficult one. Doctors are trained in differential diagnosis, whereby they practice identifying a single disease from a list of possible choices. Based on the symptoms that are present, a doctor will choose from a list of possibilities, attempting to rule out the most serious first and proceeding from there to the more common or mundane. Autoimmune conditions tend to be lower on the list of priorities and have multiple causes that can make them more difficult to identify. Autoimmune symptoms can also be so generalized at first that they could apply to many conditions. With a low priority, multiple causes, and a variety of common symptoms, arriving at an autoimmune diagnosis can be difficult and time consuming.

When a Wrong Diagnosis Occurs

A wrong diagnosis, or diagnostic error, is not such an uncommon occurrence as one would hope it would be. International conferences are held all over the world to address this leading cause of malpractice lawsuits and enormous harm. In 1999, the Institute of Medicine estimated that up to 98,000 deaths per year occur as a result of diagnostic error. Many more go unnoticed, creating a silent epidemic of medical error in this country.

A Harvard study found that diagnostic error accounted for 17 percent of all known preventable errors. According to the CDC website, in 2009–2010, there were 1.2 billion office visits to doctors. Applying the Harvard estimate of diagnostic errors, there were over 204 million diagnostic errors in the United States for that time period.

Doctors are routinely challenged by patients, as the complexity of disease in this modern age is enormous. To correctly diagnose a patient with accuracy, a doctor would have to be familiar with anatomy, physiology, toxicology, psychology, endocrinology, neurology, immunology, cardiology, orthopedics, diet and nutrition, and so on. Most doctors are familiar with anatomy and addressing symptoms through medication protocols. This creates a large gap in knowledge that often leads to a missed or wrong diagnosis.

QUESTION

Who is the best doctor to see if I think that I have an autoimmune condition?
There is no dedicated field of autoimmunity at the moment in the medical profession. Each area of medicine has doctors who specialize in certain autoimmune conditions. Depending on your symptoms, consult the appropriate doctor, or ask for a referral. Examples are a neurologist for the nerves; a rheumatologist for joints; an endocrinologist for hormones; and a gastroenterologist for digestion.

Autoimmune diseases are a good example of this. Knowledge of anatomy is helpful, but physiology explains more about what's happening within the body between various cells, tissues, organs, and systems. In order to have the best chance of achieving a correct diagnosis in this area, the doctor needs to be familiar with physiology, immunology, toxicology, psychology, nutrition, and laboratory testing.

Physiology

Physiology helps explain the nuts and bolts of how everything is functioning or not functioning. How a chemical affects the physiology is important to know. If the cell-to-cell response to chemicals is not known, as it isn't in over 99 percent of cases, then knowing how chemical toxins can impact tissues, organs, and even symptoms can help to provide important clues. When physiology is not understood, knowing how to treat a condition is less likely to be successful.

A good example of this takes place when acid reflux is present in the body. Most people, including doctors, have been educated by pharmaceutical company television ads to assume that this is caused by excess amounts of HCL. The medical treatment is to take medications that lower levels of HCL in the body.

For decades, however, holistic healthcare practitioners have known that acid reflux is caused by low levels of HCL in the stomach that leads to cycles of overproduction and underproduction of acid. During the overproduction cycles, the common symptoms associated with acid reflux are present, but it is the constantly low levels of HCL that create the problem. Holistic doctors have had great success when increasing the levels of HCL to restore balance.

ALERT

Don't be afraid to work with both conventional and alternative healthcare practitioners. Each can provide a point of view that might not be considered by the other. Although it can cost more to use both, it can also produce the best results in the shortest amount of time.

If HCL levels remain low, or suppressed as with antacid medications, physiology tells us that the patient can suffer a long list of ailments and loss of nutrients such as calcium, magnesium, zinc, iron, B_{12}, folic acid, and the proteins necessary to support health and balance in the body. Decreased absorption of iron, zinc, and protein can paralyze the immune system. Currently, only calcium loss is seen as a slight possibility in HCL deficiencies by the medical field. Knowledge of physiology creates greater understanding and comprehension.

Immunology

Knowledge of immunology specifically helps identify how the immune system responds to various challenges and how those responses can play a role in the development of autoimmunity. Even the simpler categories of knowing whether Th1, Th2, or Th17 immune cells might respond under certain conditions can help narrow the diagnosis.

Understanding immune system function is very important in knowing when an autoimmune condition is present or might be in the process of developing. Like every other system in the body, however, it is intricately connected to the other systems, so knowledge of them all and how they function in autoimmunity can be very helpful.

Toxicology

Environmental impact can be a monstrous giant to deal with when there are well over 650,000 chemicals in the U.S. workplace alone. Difficulty is added by the 10,000-plus chemicals added to foods, the effects of medication, and so forth. Toxicology effects can vary by race, gender, and lifestyle. Careful consideration of general exposures, past and present, along with transgenerational influences, can help identify added risks.

ESSENTIAL

Make your home a safe haven by reducing your exposure to chemicals as much as possible. This can include eating organic, free-range foods and extend to use of HEPA air filters, water and shower filters, non-toxic detergents, soaps, and conditioners. It's much easier to regulate toxin exposures in the home than it is in the world.

The complexity of this area alone requires that a physician take all the time necessary to carefully arrive at the right diagnosis.

Psychology

One of the most common responses that patients hear when a doctor is not able to discover what's responsible for their symptoms or conditions is that "it's all in your head." It would probably be better if that were true, as it would make coming up with the correct diagnosis a bit easier. That's not the case, however. A large percentage of diseases are considered to have stress and psychological influences as causes or cofactors. Unfortunately, medicine created separation between mind and body decades ago, which leads to a great many misunderstandings and incomplete assessments.

Nutrition

Nutrition can be a very important consideration in any diagnosis. Every cell requires nutrients in order to maintain normal function. Inadequate levels of nutrients in the diet or the rapid usage of nutrients resulting from disease states and excess levels of inflammation can lead to nutrient deficiencies very quickly. Most medical schools, however, only teach 2–70 hours of nutrition, creating a huge gap in the knowledge and understanding of the body as it relates to nutrients. Too little, and sometimes too much, of any one nutrient can have a major impact on immune system function.

FACT

In her book *The Wahls Protocol*, Terry Wahls, MD, provides details on how she used diet and nutrition to create a spontaneous remission of her multiple sclerosis symptoms. By focusing on supplying the cells with the nutrients they need, she was able to go from being wheelchair bound to walking, swimming, and biking.

Arriving at a correct diagnosis with autoimmune conditions is a challenging task in modern medicine. Most doctors are ill-equipped to undertake such a task. Specialists are often consulted, but they are limited in their breadth of knowledge, although highly specialized within narrow fields. You should persist in consulting doctors until you are satisfied that your concerns have been addressed and that all choices have been considered.

Laboratory Testing

Laboratory testing is one of the common approaches that most doctors use to confirm the presence or absence of disease processes and progression in the body. Certain lab tests can help determine whether a disease or imbalance might be present. Most doctors start with a basic blood test called a complete blood count with differential, combined with a comprehensive metabolic panel. This provides the essential basic information on certain red and white blood cells as well as nutrients, hormones, and other factors. With autoimmune issues, however, a doctor should not stop there, as this type of testing is not specific enough.

Antibody Testing

Antibodies are one of the primary responses associated with autoimmune diseases. There are several antibody tests available that cover such conditions as thyroid, Lyme, and celiac diseases. The general antibody test that is used most often is the antinuclear antibody (ANA) test. This is positive in several diseases and is a good indicator of autoimmune conditions.

Immunoglobulin Testing

Immunoglobulins are technically antibodies produced in response to antigens that generate immune responses in autoimmune diseases and other conditions. There are five main immunoglobulins (Ig) that are tested for, which include IgA (mucous membranes), IgG (past infections), IgM (current infections), IgE (allergies and parasites), and IgD (unknown).

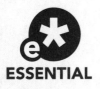

ESSENTIAL

Test results are just one part of the equation that helps determine whether a person has an autoimmune condition. All test results require interpretation and by themselves tend not to be too reliable. Often a test result will require that more tests be done, so don't be alarmed by any one test finding.

Immunoglobulins can help point to a better understanding of the cause, duration, and tissues involved in an autoimmune response.

C-Reactive Protein and Homocysteine

These two blood markers help indicate increased levels of inflammation in the body. They have been associated with Alzheimer's, cancers, and cardiovascular diseases.

Blood Sugar Testing

Blood sugar levels are commonly tested in the comprehensive metabolic panel, but it is not a very accurate indication of blood sugar regulation in the body. More specific markers include the hemoglobin A1c, which reveals the average blood sugar level for the past 90 days, and the oral glucose tolerance test, which indicates how well your body responds to sugar. Fructosamine is another test that only measures blood sugar levels over the past 2–3 weeks, but it is rarely used by most doctors.

Heavy Metals

Heavy metals are one of the common environmental toxins associated with autoimmune diseases and testing for heavy metals can provide a valuable piece of information that should always be considered in autoimmunity, but seldom is. Mercury, lead, cadmium, and aluminum are common heavy metals that can show up with autoimmune diseases. Gold has even been implicated in some instances.

FACT

Gold has been used in anti-inflammatory medications to treat rheumatoid arthritis and other autoimmune conditions for over eighty years. Its use, however, can also lead to the development of autoimmune kidney conditions, such as autoimmune thrombocytopenia and glomerulonephritis.

Gold and mercury are two heavy metals that are sometimes used in medications. Their use in drugs has been linked to causing several types of autoimmune diseases, especially those involving the kidneys.

Hormone Testing

Estrogen has a high correlation with autoimmune diseases, but other hormones such as testosterone, progesterone, pregnenolone, and especially thyroid hormones are also involved. Getting your hormones tested can help to more clearly indicate if hormones are a part of the problem and need to be addressed.

Nutrients

Nutrient deficiencies are often a factor in autoimmune diseases and can predispose an individual to increased risk of not only one condition, but several. Zinc and vitamin D are two of the main deficiencies found in autoimmune disease and immune system dysregulation. Vitamin A and B deficiencies are also commonly present.

Misunderstood Autoimmune Conditions

Autoimmune conditions can be misdiagnosed, mistreated, or missed altogether. Any condition that causes runaway inflammation in the body could end up causing conditions that look and act like an autoimmune response. The tissues could be attacked directly, or simply be a bystander damaged by high levels of chronic inflammation. Knowing which process is taking place can help determine the best treatment choice.

Direct Attack

How many doctors does it take to diagnose autoimmune disease? With the body attacking and damaging itself during autoimmune diseases, these conditions may look like any number of possibilities. Take lupus for example. It can damage various tissues and organs, such as the skin, joints, lungs, heart, brain, or kidneys. Initially, it might look like just a skin problem, or just arthritis, or a kidney disease when damaging the kidneys. A person could end up going to a skin doctor, rheumatologist, or internist at various stages of the disease. The whole picture may not become clear for years.

Consider the case of a patient who suffered from arthritic pain for 20 years before being correctly diagnosed. During that time, she had visited thirteen doctors and was told that she had a variety of conditions ranging from carpal tunnel to bursitis to the flu. Finally, a doctor took some x-rays and knew right away that it was rheumatoid arthritis. This was confirmed with blood work.

ALERT

A busy doctor may not take the time needed to arrive at the correct diagnosis. It's important to continue to look for answers, even when doctors think they know or don't know. If your condition continues to worsen, or won't go away, consult with a specialist to see if further testing is warranted.

RightDiagnosis.com states that autoimmune adrenal conditions such as Addison's disease and Cushing's syndrome are often misdiagnosed as depression or schizophrenia. Someone might be treated with antidepressants and drugs for schizophrenia for years before the correct condition is discovered.

Innocent Bystander

Anything that creates high levels of inflammation can damage tissues. Systemic candida infections are a good example. Candida is linked to over 120 conditions, mostly by way of it promoting high levels of inflammation in the body. Many of those conditions are autoimmune conditions. Another way candida creates inflammation is through a cell wall protein found in candida that is identical to the gliadin protein in gluten. The body responds to the presence of both with high levels of inflammation.

Gluten is often linked to several autoimmune diseases. The levels of inflammation associated with gluten could result in conditions of the digestive tract such as inflammatory bowel disease (IBD) and Crohn's, or tissues farther away, such as with multiple sclerosis affecting the brain and spinal cord.

How Autoimmune Treatments Can Worsen Your Condition

The goal of medical treatment is to control or reverse symptoms of diseases. Causes are usually too complicated to address in medicine, so the focus is on managing the symptoms. If a disease process can be slowed down and the patient can extend his life by days, weeks, months, or years, the treatments are generally considered a success. The fact that a disease will continue to progress is not taken into consideration as part of a successful outcome.

QUESTION

Will prescription medications address the root cause of my condition? Doctors are able to treat some things, as when they use antibiotics to treat bacterial infections, but the underlying cause that allowed the infection to exist is not addressed. Medical doctor Mark Hyman states, "doctors are very well trained to treat symptoms and diseases, but *not* to address the underlying imbalances that perpetuate illness."

Drugs are one of the main treatments used in medicine to treat all diseases. They are powerful chemicals designed to create a proven outcome with some degree of certainty, as demonstrated through testing and clinical trials. How they create their desired effect specifically is usually not known and opens the door to hundreds of other possible results, called side effects. The average number of side effects per medication is in the neighborhood of 400. This speaks to the powerful nature of the chemicals that make up drugs.

Known

Some drugs are known to cause autoimmune conditions. Antibiotics like doxycycline, minocycline, and rifampin, cholesterol-lowering drugs like Lipitor and Zocor, and even autoimmune drugs like Remicade are all known to cause autoimmune diseases. Immunosuppressant drugs can lead to increased risks of infections and cause severe side effects. Chemotherapy drugs are being used more with autoimmune conditions and bring with them a long list of harmful side effects. These powerful drugs often require frequent monitoring to ensure that they aren't creating other diseases and complications.

Unknown

One of the leading causes of autoimmunity, or its exacerbation, is the environment. The number of chemicals and heavy metals present in the body are constantly challenging humans via internal and external exposures. Managing such exposures is very tricky as they are usually taking place on an ongoing basis, directly or indirectly. Compounding the risk of these exposures is the fact that medications are present in the environment.

ALERT

Thousands of tons of pharmaceuticals are released into the environment every year. Wastewater treatment plants are unable to filter out these compounds and they end up being dumped into the environment, affecting the wildlife and health of people in the vicinity of the plants. Many of these compounds end up in household tap water.

The United States Geological Survey organization estimates that over 80 percent of the waterways in the United States are contaminated with pharmaceutical residues. These drugs enter the waterways via excretion by humans and animals, and by disposal of medications by hospitals and other facilities. The most popular drugs tend to be found in the highest concentrations. As much as 93 percent of the drugs that enter our waterways are able to pass through unaffected by community filtration systems and enter the environment and tap water. The inability to filter out such drugs means that everyone and the environment is being exposed to small amounts of drugs on a daily basis.

In the past, it was thought that it took large exposures to chemicals to cause disease. This is now known to be untrue as even minute amounts can create problems. The field of nanomedicine shows that the smallest doses can actually create significant effects. These drugs can exacerbate autoimmune diseases in millions of people worldwide without them ever having been directly exposed to the drugs.

Chasing Symptoms Instead of the Cause

Every diagnosis carries with it a set of signs and symptoms that are more or less particular to a certain disease. While signs are considered something that a doctor or observer would notice, and symptoms are what the patient experiences, they are usually lumped together and referred to as symptoms.

The symptoms presented in every case will have varying degrees of specificity, with some being more general and others more specific to the condition present.

ESSENTIAL

The body has a great ability to adapt to many symptoms. When that adaptation no longer works, or feedback pathways are no longer functioning, diseases can progress without producing many symptoms. The first symptoms of a heart attack are usually the attack itself. Symptomless conditions are often referred to as silent killers.

Nonspecific symptoms can include body aches, weakness, and fatigue. Specific symptoms can include fevers that indicate an infection, or swelling around a joint or tissue that indicates a physical injury. Many conditions share similar symptoms that make one condition look like another. This makes an accurate diagnosis often difficult to achieve. Further evaluation via testing to determine exact causes is often needed.

Since symptoms are the guideposts by which a diagnosis is made, they also tend to be the measure of how successful any treatment is. This is problematic in that symptoms are just a signal from the body that something is in a state of imbalance or dysfunction. Like a ringing doorbell that tells you that someone is ringing the bell but doesn't tell you who or what is ringing the bell, a symptom is merely an indicator of some imbalance but doesn't tell you much about it. If you disconnect the bell and someone tries to ring the doorbell, nothing will happen that lets you know that someone is trying to get your attention. That doesn't mean that there is no one at the door, only that you are not aware of it any longer. Symptoms are feedback that the body provides so that you may properly address the cause. If the feedback is suppressed, as with medications, or absent, due to a breakdown in the body's ability to alert you, disease progresses uninterrupted.

Some diseases are like this in that they can develop slowly and progress through several stages until they become a full-blown disease. Without being able to recognize them, how can we appropriately address them?

Symptoms of Disease

Symptoms of disease can vary according to the tissues, organs, or systems being affected. Inflammation is often present, but that alone is not very specific, as it can be expected to occur with most disease processes. Fevers indicate infections. Gas, bloating, and diarrhea can indicate digestive system imbalances. Headaches and tremors can indicate nervous system disorders. All of these can be involved in autoimmune conditions depending on where they take place.

FACT

Pandemic and epidemic diseases are rare these days. The Black Death (an epidemic of bubonic plague) and the Spanish flu (an influenza pandemic) together killed about 80 million people worldwide within a few years. In comparison, modern diseases like malaria and AIDS kill about 3 million a year. Improvements in sanitation have played a big role in lessening global diseases.

With any disease, there can be acute symptoms and chronic symptoms. Acute symptoms can be more pronounced and stand out more initially, whereas chronic symptoms may come and go over time with varying degrees of intensity. The body can initially respond very strongly, but may wear out through prolonged stress and damage and produce fewer symptoms later. Although not often considered, a lack of symptoms can be a sign that something is wrong as well. Paying attention to your body can help you to recognize early symptoms. Keeping a written record of these can be very helpful later.

Symptoms of Healing

There are many symptoms that can indicate healing, but for various reasons you might mistake them as being a sign of a disease or some other imbalance. The immune system, for example, often produces an inflammatory response as part of the healing process. With inflammation, you can experience aches, pains, fevers, and fatigue. Although this is a healthy response and one that you would expect to see, most people identify it as a sign of sickness. Allowing the body to go through this healing process, however, instead of interfering with it, can help strengthen the body and the immune system, as happens with children growing up. Interfering with it may mean that the immune system never gets to develop fully. This is a key component of the hygiene hypothesis, which states that the immune system needs to be challenged in order to develop healthy responses.

In general, as symptoms lessen and resolve themselves, and energy levels improve, healing is considered to be taking place, and all is well. In holistic philosophies, the body is known to go through a retracing process whereby symptoms may appear to get worse before they get better as the body goes through the process of rebuilding and repair.

ALERT

Retracing is also known as healing reactions, healing crisis, and flare-ups. A flare-up is also a term commonly used with autoimmune diseases to describe a reccurrence of symptoms. Both incidences describe the reappearance of symptoms, one moving toward health and one moving away from health.

Consulting with a holistic healthcare provider can help to correctly identify which path your body is on. In general, holistic healthcare providers focus on the patient and restoring health, while medical doctors focus on controlling disease.

Spontaneous Remission: When Unexpected Improvement Occurs

The 1993 publication of *Spontaneous Remission: An Annotated Bibliography* by authors Carlyle Hirshberg and Brendan O'Regan looked at 3,500 cases of spontaneous healing that occurred in people from around the world. By combing through 800 journals in 20 different languages, they collected evidence of the reversibility of disease in various illnesses from cancer and autoimmune diseases, to diabetes, bone fractures, and a variety of simple and severe conditions.

Although most doctors are witness to these types of healings, they are rarely recorded and often dismissed as mistakes in diagnosis and lab findings. Most doctors by and large aren't even interested in finding out what caused these cures to take place. The statement that patients commonly hear is, "I don't know what you're doing, but whatever it is, keep doing it." This under-reporting is common and does little to advance our understanding of the true nature of humans when it comes to healing.

QUESTION

Are there any diseases or conditions that are incurable?
There are many diseases and conditions that are thought to be incurable by mainstream medicine, but for which there is evidence of people being cured through the use of prayer, vitamins, herbs, diet, or meditation. The field of epigenetics explains how genes can be activated or turned off, depending on the influence of the environment around them.

Authors Hirshberg and O'Regan found cases in which "terminally ill" patients, suffering from "incurable" diseases, were cured without medical treatment, or by treatments deemed to be incapable of producing a cure. This pattern repeated itself over and over again in the studies that they evaluated.

Other authors use different words to identify these healings, as they don't believe that they occurred just out of the blue. Dr. Kelly Turner uses the phrase "radical remission" and has written a book by the same name. She identifies nine factors that play a role in creating these remissions:

1. Changing your diet
2. Taking charge of your health
3. Following your intuition
4. Using herbs and supplements
5. Releasing suppressed emotions
6. Increasing positive emotions
7. Embracing social support
8. Deepening your spiritual connection
9. Having strong reasons to live

Some of these factors are echoed in the work of Dr. Moshe Frenkel, who calls these remissions exceptional. He emphasizes establishing connections to God and the people around you. He also says, "We need to nurture our own 'soil'—our bodies." Additional components of his approach include supplements, homeopathy, diet, and exercise. Connecting to others and the use of supplements are suggested in both approaches and in many of the approaches often used by holistic healthcare practitioners.

Most importantly, taking charge of your own health is a key factor in creating spontaneous remission in autoimmune disease. You know yourself best, and you alone have the power to make the changes that you need to make in your life to achieve greater health. Autoimmunity is life out of balance. Bringing balance back to your life is an important part of any healing process.

CHAPTER 5

Mindful Steps for Healing

Intention, determination, attitude, self-reflection, and purpose are all useful keys in creating a successful approach to healing the mind and body. Each of these describes an approach in which the mind is central to the process. Alone and collectively, they have been used for centuries to create health, abundance, prosperity, and happiness. Each one is a process whereby the mind influences your behaviors and your body, as though the mind and body are separate. Science is only beginning to reveal how intricately intertwined the mind and body are, so much so that they should always be considered as a united whole.

Common Medical Mistakes in Treating Autoimmune Disease

The human body is an amazingly complex organism that science and medicine are still attempting to decipher and understand. So great is its complexity that the study of the body is divided into the various organs and systems in order to make studying them easier. This artificial separation of the body into various parts, however, can create problems when trying to understand the human body as a whole. Instead of simplifying the understanding of the body, it can have the opposite effect and further distance us from the entire truth of what's taking place.

The complexity of the human body is so incomprehensible that some people call it intelligent design, the scientific proof of God or some higher agency. Central to the idea of intelligent design is the concept of irreducible complexity, whereby a system so intricately connected can cease functioning effectively by removal of any one part. The body is not just one complex system, but many.

The study of autoimmunity highlights this problematic segmentation and dissociation. Instead of one field of autoimmunity, we have multiple fields of specialties within medicine wherein each one deals with the respective autoimmune conditions that come under its umbrella. A unified, whole approach and combined knowledge of the common factors present in autoimmunity is lacking. This attempt to simplify our understanding of the body has created walls that some specialists are unable to see past, and specialty languages that need to be translated into a broader, more comprehensive picture.

This segmented approach created a tragic error when mind and body were separated into the fields of medicine and psychotherapy. Medical doctors were charged with caring for the physical body, while psychiatrists and psychologists were charged with handling mental/emotional conditions. Separating the body this way into physical and psychological components created a huge chasm in our understanding of the body as a whole.

The Physical

The physical body is the nuts and bolts of medicine. From the medical perspective, it is a finite collection of organs and tissues that can be dissected down to the smallest cells.

Medicine often views this physical body as imperfect, requiring constant intervention. As long as the parts haven't worn out, it can be taken apart and put back together like a car. Like a house, it can be hammered, sawed, nailed, and hinged together, and when the real materials aren't available, substitute materials made of plastic and metal will do. The truth of this comparison is found in the surgeon's toolbox, which isn't that much different from a carpenter's or a mechanic's toolbox.

The Medical Approach

The medical doctor sees her role as righting the body's wrong. She is providing medical intervention to correct an imperfect design. Although medicine doesn't actually understand autoimmunity yet, it treats it as best as it can. Based on the information that is known to date, doctors create and follow protocols that they hope might be useful. Typically, a doctor uses medications to address the symptoms, even though medications are frequently known to create imbalances within the body. Using this approach, the medical prognosis is that once a person has an autoimmune condition, she will always have it.

ALERT

The practice of medicine is often seen as an art form as much as it is a science-based trade. Each doctor is like an artist with a different point of view and understanding and interpretation of the facts. This creates a lot of variability from one doctor to another and becomes a good reason for getting second and third opinions on anything concerning your health.

If the medicines aren't effective for the physical symptoms, then the cause will be deemed to be a psychological problem requiring a separate approach to address issues of the mind. Unfortunately, medications are once again often the only choice offered, and often with hefty side effects such as suicidal thoughts and ideation.

The Holistic Approach

The holistic doctor sees his role as aiding the body to do that which it knows how to do. By addressing the person and not the symptoms, it seeks to improve function by providing the necessary building blocks for health and the correct environment to further facilitate healing. A holistic doctor will use a wide variety of tools to address a wide variety of causes. Diet, supplements, detoxification, exercise, meditation, prayer, and other modalities assist the body in regaining health and vibrancy. The goal of the holistic practitioner is nothing less than 100 percent health. It views mind and body as one integrated whole. Understanding what creates health is more important than simply suppressing the symptoms of disease.

QUESTION

Are holistic medicine and complementary and alternative medicine (CAM) the same thing?
Holistic therapies have been around for thousands of years, while CAM has only been around since the early to mid-nineteenth century. In general, CAM is the adoption of holistic therapies such as acupuncture, homeopathy, herbs, supplements, and mind-body approaches along with traditional medical practices. An increasing number of doctors are turning to science-based holistic therapies in order to assist patients more effectively.

A holistic practitioner would consider that if the approach being used isn't working to restore health, then the approach is wrong, the understanding of what's taking place is faulty, or the substances being used are ineffective. Reconsideration of everything is needed in order to achieve better results. Acceptance of an ineffective approach and continued use of that approach does little to serve the patient.

The Psychological

The field of psychotherapy in Western medicine is firmly rooted in the separation of mind and body. Unlike Eastern medicine, in which the two are still considered as a whole, Western medicine delegates issues of the mind to the psychiatrist and psychologist. This act of separation has produced limited benefits, while also creating a great number of misperceptions and misunderstandings.

When a doctor tells a patient that her troubles are all in her head, it can be a crushing assessment in which the patient is labeled as having no "real" condition that medicine can help her with. This patient will be banished to the realms of psychiatric illness and the stigma that often goes with it. Talk therapy and medications are the primary tools of modern psychotherapy. A psychiatrist, who is a medical doctor, will address psychotherapeutic conditions primarily as a biochemical imbalance of the nervous system and prescribe drugs in an attempt to balance the system and stop the symptoms.

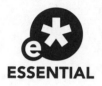

ESSENTIAL

The use of pastors and priests as counselors and therapists is a centuries old practice that continues to this day. Only in a few states are they required to hold a separate license in order to provide counseling services. Those who don't charge a fee for these services don't generally need to hold a license.

A psychologist, on the other hand, isn't usually able to write prescriptions and uses various talk or cognitive therapies to help resolve issues. Both address autoimmunity through their respective approaches and both have seen limited success. A 2003 study in the *Journal of Clinical Psychiatry* noted that nearly two-thirds of patients receive no benefit for depression when using medications. As the former head of research for the pharmaceutical company GlaxoSmithKline, Allen Roses, MD, stated, "The vast majority of drugs only work in 30 or 50 percent of the people." Drugs are obviously not the final solution.

The understanding of any one area of the body will always be incomplete until we understand the body as a whole, where mind and body are one. Attempting to understand the complete picture via psychology faces the same type of fragmentation, as differing approaches compete with one another.

Old-World Psychotherapy

Much of science, medicine, and therefore public perception, is stuck in an old model of understanding psychotherapy. Psychotherapy in this perspective focuses on "mental" illnesses in which reality plays no role. Anyone with a "psychological" problem is headed for disaster unless they can snap out of it. All hope for a cure lies in being able to help the patient realize that his thinking is amiss and that correct thinking will cure the problem. Talk therapy can help the patient to release old beliefs and understand why his thoughts were off.

Present-Day Psychotherapy

Present-day psychotherapy is still influenced heavily by old-world psychology. Newer approaches look at the influence of genetics and even epigenetics. Physical imbalances in how the nerves function and communicate can create psychological imbalances. Psychoneuroimmunology and biological psychiatry are two of the modern advancements in psychology that are helping to provide important information in the area of autoimmunity.

Psychoneuroimmunology, a term coined in 1975 by Robert Ader, looks at how stress and trauma can affect the immune and nervous systems. Discoveries in this field have done a lot to improve our understanding of the mind-body connection. Studies in this area provide insights into autoimmune conditions and their relationship to stress and emotions.

ALERT

Psychiatric medications are powerful drugs that shouldn't be shared with others, as often happens with some drugs such as antibiotics. Common adverse events include stroke, seizures, tremors, confusion, sudden cardiac failure, and possible death. Antidepressants are commonly associated with suicidal behavior.

Biological psychiatry looks at how imbalances in the function of nerves contribute to mental conditions. Unfortunately, most of the work in this area is for drug development, which hasn't been as successful as hoped for when dealing with autoimmune conditions.

New-World Psychotherapy

New-world psychotherapy is beginning to take root and demonstrate its value in developing therapies in the area of mind-body medicine.

Foundational to this evolving psychotherapy is the recognition that mind and body are not separate parts, but unified, and intricately so. Biology is behavior and behavior is biology. Both are constantly affecting each other and creating your thoughts, emotions, and outlook on life. Somatic Experiencing and Trauma Release Exercises are two examples of new therapies that create effective changes in this area. Somatic Experiencing is a psychobiological method for resolving trauma symptoms and relieving chronic stress, while Trauma Release Exercises are a series of exercises that assist the body in releasing deep muscular patterns of stress, tension and trauma.

The Mind-Body Connection in Autoimmunity

Mind-body medicine is a rapidly emerging field, as continued treatment failures in Western medicine and successes in other healthcare fields drive the need for a better approach to healing. Holistic healthcare practitioners have explored the mind-body connection for centuries. Eastern medicine practitioners have found it to be an essential component when addressing both the physical and psychological aspects of health. In holistic healing circles, any approach that doesn't take into consideration both mind and body is destined for limited results and failure.

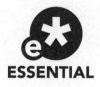

ESSENTIAL

Traditional Chinese medicine (TCM) and Ayurvedic medicine have both incorporated the use of mind-body medicine for thousands of years. In both practices, specific organs of the body are associated with specific emotions, such as liver/anger. In this context, anger could cause imbalances of the liver, and liver conditions could lead to states of anger. Many holistic methods have adopted these organ and emotion relationships.

Research has shown that one can expect exacerbation of autoimmune conditions due to the effects of stress. A 2004 study in the journal *Psychosomatic Medicine* on the effects of stress on patients with lupus found an increase in subjective symptoms and inflammatory markers in the blood from daily stress.

In the field of psychoneuroimmunology, stress-induced dysregulation of the immune system has been shown to increase symptoms of inflammation. While short-term stress can help protect the body by accelerating immune repair in cases of tissue damage, long-term, chronic stress turns potentially beneficial effects into harmful effects.

Over 300 studies have been done on the effects of stress on the immune system. These studies show how various psychological events can alter immune system function in ways that dysregulate immune responses excessively, up or down. Central to the degree of stress someone experiences is how each person may perceive stress or respond to it. How one perceives stressful events is often influenced by how doctors and healthcare practitioners relate information to their patients. These effects are known as the placebo and nocebo effects, and can affect both the physical and the psychological aspects of health.

Placebo Effect

The placebo effect is one of the most easily recognizable areas of mind-body medicine. It is commonly described as the positive result that a patient receives when he believes that something or someone can help him. If a healthcare practitioner tells a patient that he will overcome his illness and regain his health, the patient is much more likely to do this. Regardless of the substance being used to treat him, or the person treating him, if the patient believes that he will be healed, it is more likely to happen. A placebo can be effective as much as 50 percent of the time or more.

ALERT

Placebos have been used in medicine for centuries. Doctors have used sugar pills, bread pills, colored water, and other substances with great success. Recent research out of Harvard University indicates that while a placebo may make a person feel better, it may not actually change any of the physical findings in the body. It's important to pay attention to blood work and lab results, even when feeling better.

The placebo effect is so effective that when patients are told they are receiving a placebo treatment, they receive twice as much symptom relief as patients who receive no treatment. Ted Kaptchuk, Harvard Medical School faculty member and director of the Program in Placebo Studies, has shown that even when the treatment is fake, patients do better when the doctor spends more time with them.

Placebos are commonly used in testing drugs, when a drug is tested against a sugar pill. The participants receiving each substance are not told which one is which and they believe that they are receiving the drug in both instances. The gold standard in clinical testing is the double-blind, randomized, placebo-controlled study. Any drug that makes it to market is supposed to go through this rigorous testing protocol. Unfortunately for many drugs, they are not able to beat the placebo effect, and so pharmaceutical companies are trying to do away with the placebo component in drug testing. Opponents point out that if a drug can't beat a sugar pill, then it should not be approved, especially given the number of side effects that go along with each drug.

Nocebo Effect

The nocebo effect is the opposite of the placebo effect. It is the dark side of the mind-body connection. If someone believes that she will get sick, then she is likely to get sick. Robert A. Hahn, PhD, reports that studies have shown instances when surgical patients who expect to die on the operating table, do so.

The ability to create negative effects in patients by what a doctor says has been called "Voodoo Death" by researchers who cite the 1942 article of the same name by Walter B. Cannon. The paper highlights how a person's cultural beliefs can induce disease and death. In the voodoo culture, the witch doctor's words carry the most weight. In hospital cultures, the medical doctors' words carry the most weight.

Harvard researcher Ted Kaptchuk has shown that when patients are told to expect certain side effects from their treatments, they manifest them. Lissa Rankin, MD, calls this medical hexing. In an article in *Psychology Today*, Dr. Rankin states, "Every time your doctor tells you you have an 'incurable' illness or that you'll be on medication for the rest of your life or that you have a 5 percent five-year survival, they're essentially cursing you with a form of 'medical hexing.'

Together, the placebo and nocebo effects create physiological and psychological effects in the mind-body mechanism that reinforce our beliefs about health and illness. What a person believes may be as important a factor in treating autoimmunity as anything else.

Meditation, Prayer, and Mindfulness

Examples of the effectiveness of mind-body medicine have been with us for centuries. Meditation, prayer, and mindfulness are three of the most familiar forms that most people cite in this area.

Prayer

Of all the mind-body approaches to healing, prayer is one of the oldest. It is believed to have been around since the earliest humans. Whether it is a spoken invocation, a sung verse, or even a dance, prayer has been credited with saving lives and curing autoimmune diseases, among many other forms of disease. As much as the physical and psychological have been separated for decades, spirituality is even more separated due to science's reluctance to study its effects.

QUESTION

Has prayer been shown to affect the immune system?
Scientists at Oral Roberts University found that prayer can increase immune system function by 35–40 percent by causing the brain to release chemicals that act on the immune system.

Prayer fulfills one of the common tenets of healing and spontaneous remissions in that it demonstrates the social support that people receive from members of their spiritual affiliations. It also connects people to a higher purpose that gives people meaning and purpose to their lives. Social support along with meaning and purpose are mentioned as ways to create spontaneous remissions by author Kelly Turner, PhD, in her book, *Radical Remission*.

In her book *The How of Happiness*, Sonja Lyubomirsky states that "almost seven out of ten Americans report praying every single day, and only 6 percent report never praying." Such overwhelming numbers of people lend weight to the validity of prayer's effectiveness in many people's lives.

Meditation

Meditation, like prayer, is a centuries-old practice. It has its roots in many religious practices and is often associated with longer periods of inner focus that help create relaxation and improve health, among other attributes. Meditation may involve repetition of certain phrases or maintenance of various body postures. It is often associated with the practice of yoga, although its practice is more universal.

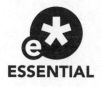

ESSENTIAL

Meditation is credited with many amazing feats. Indian mystics, Tibetan Buddhist monks, and ascetic Hindus are all credited with mastering meditation to the point that they can defy many known physical laws. Fire-walking is a common feat that thousands of people have accomplished through self-help and self-empowerment seminars around the world, highlighting the power of the mind.

Meditation has been shown to reverse the effects of stress in people's lives, especially when stress affects immune system function. Researchers in Norway showed that meditation can lessen the pro-inflammatory effects of stress on the immune system. Where stress revs up the nervous and immune systems, meditation can quiet them both down. Researchers from Spain looked at transcendental meditation and found that "the technique of meditation studied seems to have a significant effect on immune cells, manifesting in the different circulating levels of lymphocyte subsets analyzed."

Mindfulness

Mindfulness meditation is one of the most studied forms of meditation today. It focuses on creating complete awareness of the present moment without judging or reacting to it. This can be accomplished by focusing on the movement of the breath, in and out.

Universities such as the University of California, Los Angeles, have research centers devoted to the study of mindfulness. Mindfulness-based interventions are being used in homes, schools, workplaces, and military settings with increasing frequency.

Researchers from Scotland and France found that mindfulness interventions had positive effects on quality of life in autoimmune multiple sclerosis. Researchers from the University of Wisconsin–Madison found that mindfulness-based stress reduction helped decrease post-stress inflammatory response and posit that it "may be of therapeutic benefit in chronic inflammatory conditions." Researchers at UCLA found that mindfulness meditation helps decrease the drop in the immune cells of HIV patients. Study participants who practiced meditating more had higher white blood cell counts than those who practiced it less.

FACT

The jhanas are levels of consciousness achieved during Buddhist meditation. Prolonged periods of focused concentration can lead to trance-like states of altered consciousness, ecstasy, and rapture. Monks and gurus are believed to accomplish many incredible feats while in high levels of jhana.

In all studies of meditation, prayer, and mindfulness, the main effect of these practices appears to be their ability to counter the effects of stress. The effects of stress are so pervasive in today's world that life for many people is a continuously stressful event affecting them on a daily basis. Such an onslaught eventually takes its toll on the immune system and can contribute to autoimmune conditions. Countering not only present stress but past stress as well is a necessary component of any approach to regaining and maintaining health.

Resolving Stress, Tension, and Trauma

If there were one all-encompassing area to focus on to help handle the effects of stress on a daily basis, it would be resiliency. Resiliency enables someone to recover, adapt to, and bounce back from stress, trauma, tension, and illness. If a person doesn't have resiliency, eating organic foods and eliminating exposures to toxins may do very little to help him stay or get healthy. Conversely, someone with great resiliency may be able to eat and drink anything she desires and be as healthy as a horse.

Utilizing various mind-body tools on a daily basis can help create greater resiliency physically and mentally. The union of mind and body in approaches like yoga, tai chi, and qigong have proven their effectiveness in reducing the physical effects of stress that often lead to increased levels of inflammation and worsening of autoimmune diseases. Managing ongoing levels of daily stress is very helpful, but how does one go about resolving a lifetime of stress and its effects that are stored in the body? Fortunately, the evolution of approaches in psychotherapy and related fields are providing the answers and results that many people have been searching for. Two of the most promising new therapies are somatic experiencing and tension and trauma release exercises.

Somatic Experiencing

Somatic experiencing is described as a psychobiological approach to addressing stress and trauma. Based on the observations and experience of Dr. Peter Levine in his forty-five-plus-year practice, it encompasses many various disciplines that include neuroscience, biology, physiology, psychology, and others.

Somatic experiencing (SE) is a therapeutic approach designed to address traumatic events and stress that are stored within the body. Dr. Levine has found that "human beings are readily traumatized" and these events can produce lifelong challenges that affect many systems, including the immune system.

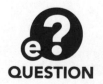

QUESTION

Can you accomplish the same results with meditation as you can with somatic experiencing?
Dr. Levine points out that meditation can be helpful, but when people have trauma stored in their body, it can be difficult to go into their inner landscape, where trauma and stress often reside. Once stored patterns of trauma and stress have been resolved, meditation can become more enjoyable and relaxed states more easily achieved.

To achieve healing and resolution of these traumas and stresses, a combination of the mind and body together is addressed in sessions with SE-trained therapists. SE helps complete unresolved traumatic and stress-induced neuromotor responses that keep people locked in patterns of anxiety, depression, fight/flight, dissociation, and withdrawal. SE often succeeds where other more conventional therapies fail.

Tension and Trauma Release Exercises

Tension and trauma release exercises (TRE) were developed by Dr. David Berceli, a trauma specialist. He created a series of exercises that assist the body in releasing deep muscular patterns of stress, tension, and trauma. Through his work and observations in war-torn countries, Dr. Berceli recognized similar patterns in how a person's body responded to trauma and stress and how natural, built-in mechanisms enabled a person to naturally resolve those events. Specific to the resolution process are the tremors and shaking that follow trauma and high levels of stress. Dr. Berceli developed a series of simple exercises that activate a process of self-induced tremors. While tremors are a natural physical response, modern medicine has misunderstood the process. Modern society often views tremors as a sign of weakness or a disease process, but when it is activated by trauma, it can be a powerful healing response that discharges overwhelming impulses to the body's nervous system. Once this process is complete, the body restores itself to a natural, integrated, and whole state.

Unlike animals, which also possess this reflex and use it to bring themselves back into balance, humans however, tend to suppress this response and end up carrying trauma and stress around inside themselves. This burden of inner trauma and stress can then play a role in autoimmune and other diseases.

ESSENTIAL

The tremors that are elicited in tension and trauma release exercises, as well as occasionally in somatic experiencing, is an unconscious process that can feel funny, strange, and foreign, as it is not under the control of the thinking mind. It generally leaves one feeling calm, relaxed, and whole.

Central to both TRE and SE is the polyvagal theory developed by Dr. Stephen Porges. The polyvagal theory states that there are two separate branches of the vagus nerve, the tenth cranial nerve. The first is a primitive branch associated with the overwhelming of the nervous system and subsequent immobilization behaviors. The second is an evolutionary advancement in humans involved with social engagement and integration. Between these is the sympathetic nervous system, which is involved in fight/flight. A person who enters a state of fight/flight can activate the primitive branch when he becomes overwhelmed by a stressful event, in which case, he doesn't return to a whole, integrated state.

This can leave people locked in a dissociated state that leads to withdrawal and the inability to regain the integrated state that leads to social engagement and a sense of wholeness. TRE resolves this polarized behavior and helps restore integration.

Supported by much of the same research as somatic experiencing, TRE often requires only one session with a trained TRE provider, although some people have been able to learn it by following Dr. Berceli's books and DVDs. Although people with more serious traumas may require follow-up sessions, most people are able to utilize TRE on their own without further supervision. TRE sessions can last as little as one minute or up to sixty minutes. They can be done in moderation (ten to twenty minutes) if you are doing them daily, or thirty to forty-five minutes if you are doing them weekly. Since the tremor mechanism has a substantial impact on the physiology of the body, you must allow for structural integration time so the body is not overwhelmed.

The TRE model is an excellent tool that anyone suffering with an autoimmune disorder can utilize daily to reduce and offset inflammation and a worsening of symptoms.

The complexity of the body requires a more whole, or holistic, and expansive appreciation of the mind and body as one. As Western medicine advances its understanding of the mind-body connection, it finds itself catching up to Eastern medicine practices that have been in place for centuries. Like mind-body medicine, together they have the greatest opportunity to assist with healing autoimmune diseases.

CHAPTER 6

Antibiotics, Candida, and the Gut

Any sound discussion of autoimmune diseases will look at the human gut and the role of this amazing ecosystem in determining health and illness in the body. Considered by some to be the densest ecosystem on the planet, the human gut is a major pathway for absorption of nutrients and elimination of toxins. As host to approximately 70 percent or more of the body's immune system and 100 trillion microbes, what happens in the gut has a significant impact on the prevention and development of autoimmune diseases.

Antibiotics: Both Cure and Curse

In 1928, Alexander Fleming made a discovery that would change the practice of medicine for decades to come when he discovered the antibiotic properties of penicillin. It wasn't until years later, however, with the assistance of Ernst Chain, Howard Florey, and the USDA's National Center for Agricultural Utilization Research Lab, that penicillin could be mass-produced and the age of antibiotics begun.

FACT

In 1945, Fleming, Chain, and Florey shared the Nobel Prize in Physiology or Medicine for the discovery of penicillin and its curative effect in various infectious diseases. All three men would also receive knighthood by the British Empire for their joint work on penicillin.

Antibiotics are credited with saving millions of lives. Prior to the development of antibiotics, the medical profession found itself unable to treat most infections successfully. People routinely died from simple infections while under medical care. Although a few antibiotics existed prior to the discovery and use of penicillin, it was the mass production and initial success of penicillin that enabled the medical field to start turning the tide against infectious diseases.

The Germ Theory and Disease

Antibiotics appeared to be the perfect answer to the theory of germs and disease as postulated by Louis Pasteur almost a century earlier. Pasteur developed the germ theory, which stated that substances too small to be seen by the naked eye were responsible for causing diseases. Prior to Pasteur's experiments, there was more focus on the environment and changes within the host as the main causes of diseases. Popular scientific opinion of his time thought that germs spontaneously appeared out of thin air. Pasteur was able to show that the germs were already present. Pasteur's germ theory gave science a more concrete enemy to focus their efforts on.

Bacteria and Other Animalcules

Pasteur's work helped expand on the work of earlier people like Antonie van Leeuwenhoek, who in the seventeenth century identified small single-celled organisms under a microscope and named them animalcules. As an amateur scientist, van Leeuwenhoek did what scientists of his time were unable to do and was the first person to see bacteria under a microscope that he made himself. These bacteria would become the primary focus of Pasteur's germ theory and the target of hundreds of antibiotics to follow.

Them or Us

Once the enemy was defined, it was established that it was them versus us, an opinion that would take decades to reverse. The use of antibiotics against bacteria and other microbes became the Holy Grail of the medical field. All bacteria were dispensable and a doctor could only do good by pre-scribing antibiotics. Every pharmaceutical company rushed to develop an army of antibiotics. With antibiotics on their side, MDs began to proclaim the end of all infectious diseases. The story would not end that way, however, as there was still much that was not yet understood about bacteria and other microbes. Perhaps if scientists had paid closer attention, they would have heeded Pasteur's earlier warning, *"Messieurs, c'est les microbes qui auront le dernier mot"* (Gentlemen, it is the microbes who will have the last word).

ESSENTIAL

Although Pasteur was credited with the germ theory, he also had great insight into the nature of microbes, or germs, as they were called back then. On his deathbed, he is credited with stating that the terrain is everything, meaning that the bacteria were most important. He also stated that "the role of the infinitely small in nature is infinitely great."

Revenge of the Bugs

Alexander Fleming was acutely aware that penicillin could create antibiotic-resistant strains of bacteria and even noted so in his Nobel Prize acceptance speech in 1945. Early on, it was apparent that antibiotic use wasn't without some risk. Antibiotics were curing people of infections, but other problems were arising from their use. Some people found themselves suffering from other conditions as a result of antibiotic use.

The Antibiotic Curse

Antibiotic resistance was a problem that soon developed after using antibiotics. It was noted that all antibiotics would have limited usefulness eventually as the bacteria they were used against had a natural ability to adapt and render the antibiotic useless. Minor infections could become major ones if antibiotics weren't used carefully. In the 1990s, authorities started warning about the end of the antibiotic era, as antibiotic resistance was now a growing concern. Shortly afterward, the World Health Organization listed antibiotic resistance as one of the top three threats to human health on the planet. It is estimated that over 2 million infections and at least 23,000 deaths each year in the United States alone are now due to antibiotic resistance, with some estimates placing that number much higher. Some sources put the yearly death total worldwide at over 2 million deaths. In 2014, Dr. Arjun Srinivasan, associate director for healthcare associated infection prevention programs at the Centers for Disease Control and Prevention in the United States, stated, "We're here. We're in the post-antibiotic era. There are patients for whom we have no therapy."

Beyond the Reach of Antibiotics

There are now over seven common species of bacteria that are beyond the reach of antibiotics. These bacteria (with tuberculosis being a main one) have developed resistance to all known antibiotics available. In some countries, over 35 percent of tuberculosis infections are antibiotic-resistant. Once antibiotics are no longer available as an option, the next choice in line, and a much more toxic one, is chemotherapy.

QUESTION

How can I tell if I have an infection that is resistant to all antibiotics?
In the United States, all doctors are supposed to test patients to check that they first have a bacterial infection, as antibiotics only work against bacteria, and then that they only prescribe an antibiotic that is proven to be effective against their specific infection. The FDA federally mandated this in 2003.

The Fungal Link

Shortly after the mass production of penicillin in 1945, it was noted that fungal candida infections were developing in people after antibiotic use. These fungal infections were beginning to be associated with other conditions like meningitis, endocarditis, and other autoimmune-type conditions like psoriasis and asthma. The rise in fungal candida research and antibiotic use has a direct correlation. A search of the U.S. National Library of Medicine shows that prior to the mass introduction of antibiotics, there were zero studies on candida in 1944. Starting with four studies in 1945, there have now been over 56,000 studies on candida since the introduction of antibiotics. In 2014 alone, there were 2,443 studies on candida. Candida has come a long way thanks to antibiotic use.

Antibiotics and LPS

Venturing out into the dark can be a risky endeavor. Not being able to see where you're going, or whether your choices are taking you in the right direction, is a recipe for disaster. The biological sciences that dominate the health fields are very much like this. They are based not on hard science (such as 1 + 1 = 2), but on soft science, in which a consensus of opinion and interpretation of "scientific" data determines current choices and practice protocols.

For decades, doctors have demonstrated a lack of understanding of how antibiotics affect the body. Often we rush to use them without considering the effects of their use on the body in ways other than we intended. Some negative effects are immediate, while others may take years to produce a noticeable effect. While "cause and effect" is easily seen in many circumstances, it is a poor model to rely on in healthcare, as some problems take years or decades to reveal themselves. In other instances, the effects seem so removed from the parts of the body typically exposed to antibiotics that a connection is not so obvious. The use of antibiotics leading to the release of lipopolysaccharides from bacteria when they are destroyed is a good example of how some antibiotic effects can be both delayed and remote from the original site of action.

Lipopolysaccharides

Lipopolysaccharides (LPS) are a combination of fats and sugars found in the cell walls of the majority of bacteria in the intestinal tract and many other tissues of the body. They help give the cell wall strength and stability, and play a role in protecting the bacteria under various conditions. Antibiotics that target the bacterial cell wall and cause the death and disintegration of the bacterial cell cause the release of lipopolysaccharides and other substances into the surrounding tissues and fluids. The human body is highly allergic to these substances and creates a strong inflammatory immune response when it senses their presence. Within reason, this response helps clean up these substances so that they don't persist in the body and cause ongoing problems.

Human Gut

The human intestinal tract is home to 100 trillion bacterial cells. These cells outnumber our own human cells by a factor of 10 to 1. With so many nonhuman cells present, it's only fitting that at least 70 percent of the body's immune system is also present in the intestinal tract to help regulate so many bacteria. Like all other types of cells in the body, bacteria have a lifespan, so one would expect to find ongoing exposure to LPS as the resident bacteria die off. The body in its infinite wisdom and design is capable of handling the daily housekeeping chores that include cleaning up a few hundred thousand, or even a million bacterial cells on a daily basis. As long as the death rate of bacteria is reasonable, there aren't going to be any issues with bacteria and LPS.

ALERT

You can help minimize the negative effects of taking antibiotics by taking probiotics at the same time. Probiotics are beneficial strains of bacteria known to colonize the intestinal tract. Take antibiotics and probiotics several hours apart from each other to avoid having the antibiotics destroy the probiotics. Use a good multistrain probiotic to achieve greater results.

A Little versus a Lot

Unfortunately, medicine treats the body more like a test tube than a complex system of interdependent tissues and cells. If bacteria are present and causing an infection, just pour some antibiotics into the tube and destroy all the bacteria. Once the bacteria are dead, the problems will go away. Antibiotics however, create a unique problem in that a five or seven-day dosage of antibiotics can wipe out practically all the bacteria in the body. This causes levels of bacterial cell death that the body wasn't designed to handle. As the bacteria hemorrhage their internal components out into the surrounding tissues, the body's housekeeping abilities quickly become overwhelmed. The subsequent levels of inflammation that are generated as a part of the body's immune system response start creating other problems.

LPS Equals Inflammation

The body's response to the presence of LPS leads to the creation of strong inflammatory cascades by stimulating pro-inflammatory proteins in the body called cytokines and chemokines. These proteins go by abbreviated names like IL-6, TNF-a, COX2, IL-12, IL-13, IL-17, IL-18, IL-10, IL-9, PGE-2, IL-1ß, and many others. With massive amounts of LPS flooding the body's tissues from antibiotic use, a 10–1,000-fold increase in inflammation has been noted. One study that appeared in the *Journal of Neuroinflammation* showed that as little as 38.5 million dead bacterial cells in a 170-pound man could prime the brain for chronic inflammation. Destroying 100 trillion cells is approximately 2.5 million times more than what is necessary to create ongoing inflammation and degeneration of the brain. Once the brain has become primed for ongoing inflammation, minimal amounts of LPS present in the circulation are enough to play a role in creating autoimmune conditions like Alzheimer's, Parkinson's, and dementia.

Candida-Related Conditions

Just as antibiotics create imbalances that can lead to chronic inflammation via the destruction of bacteria and the release of LPS, antibiotics commonly lead to the development of fungal candida and the subsequent conditions that develop as a result of its presence.

Candida normally exists in the body in a yeast form. In the yeast form, it plays a role in digestion and possibly even helping to alkalize tissues. Due to the effects of antibiotics, candida will convert from its normal beneficial yeast form to the problematic fungal form known to play a role in many diseases. Once this conversion takes place, candida can escape the confinement of the intestinal tract, spread throughout the body, and establish itself in any tissue or organ. With its ability to evade and manipulate immune responses and conditions in the body, it can grow unchecked by even healthy bodies.

ESSENTIAL

Many men make the mistake of thinking that candida is an infection that affects only women. In reality, candida is blind when it comes to gender. It can affect both men and women equally. If you've had antibiotics, chances are you have a fungal candida infection. Most people are asymptomatic when it comes to candida.

There are currently over 120 symptoms and conditions that are associated with fungal candida. These range from conditions such as acne and indigestion to heart disease, obesity, and cancers. Among the known effects are autoimmune conditions such as:

- Multiple sclerosis
- Alzheimer's disease
- Psoriasis
- Eczema
- Rheumatoid arthritis
- Diabetes
- Inflammatory bowel disease
- Scleroderma
- Autoimmune polyendocrinopathy
- Hypothyroidism
- Crohn's disease
- Asthma
- Chronic fatigue syndrome (aka myalgic encephalomyelitis)
- Ulcerative colitis
- Systemic lupus erythrematosus
- Kawasaki disease

As we learn more about candida and how it affects the body, we continue to find more associations with other conditions. The ability of candida to establish itself within any environment found in the body makes it an ideal suspect in many conditions.

Inflammation and Candida

Like LPS, candida is a strong driver of inflammation in the body. They both trigger the release of some of the same pro-inflammatory cytokines and chemokines that then create and contribute to many conditions and diseases.

IL-17

One of the main drivers of inflammation during any candida infection is the body's interleukin-17 (IL-17) cytokine response. IL-17 is produced by T helper-17 immune cells, which help regulate and recruit other white blood cells to the site of an infection. To date, this appears to be the body's most effective response against candida and it is also one of the body's most pro-inflammatory immune responses. It is a two-edged sword that can help and harm the body.

QUESTION

Are there natural substances that can reduce inflammation?
Many herbs are known to reduce the pro-inflammatory effect of cytokines in the body. Two of the most potent inhibitors of inflammation are green tea and turmeric/curcumin. Others include omega-3 fatty acids and the anti-autoimmune vitamin, vitamin D.

The IL-17 response is one of the main reasons that candida is associated with so many diseases and conditions, especially the autoimmune ones. In addition to those already mentioned, IL-17 is also associated with prostatitis, depression, interstitial cystitis, sinusitis, esophagitis, and other conditions that perfectly mirror the list of over 120 candida-related conditions.

IL-1ß and IL-18

Candida's conversion from harmless yeast to pathogenic fungus stimulates the production of IL-1ß and IL-18. These interleukins are two other major pro-inflammatory cytokines that respond to candida's presence in the body and are a factor in many autoimmune conditions. In fact, autoimmune treatments that seek to suppress these cytokines leave the patient vulnerable to candida infections. When it comes to IL-1ß, Dr. Christina Zielinski states, "I am convinced that an imbalance in our microbial microflora has a decisive influence on the development of chronic inflammatory illnesses like rheumatism, Morbus Crohn and psoriasis. Our organism is composed of ten times more microbial cells than our body's own cells. Keeping this in check is not easy. Interleukin 1ß is now turning out to be a decisive molecular switch, which the microbes use to dictate between healthy or sick."

Matrix Metalloproteinases (MMPs)

This family of enzymes plays a role in tissue repair and remodeling in the body. Candida's presence causes an increase in certain members of this enzyme family that can then lead to excessive breakdown of tissues as found in conditions like arthritis and hair loss. In excessive amounts, MMPs promote a lot of inflammation in the body.

FACT

Cytokines are proteins that act as messengers between various cell types and chemokines are a type of cytokine that acts as signaling messenger to help recruit and attract the cells needed for a particular function. Immune cytokines help coordinate the appropriate immune response, and may become dysregulated in autoimmune conditions.

In regard to the cytokines, it is not yet clear as to whether the microbes are manipulating their presence and function, or our body is in charge of everything taking place. As we learn more and more about the microbiome, it seems more logical to assume that we are still playing catch-up to organisms that have survived on this planet for millions of years longer than us.

Maintaining Good Gut Health

We've come a long way from thinking that the 100 trillion microbes of the gut were disposable "bugs" to realizing that we wouldn't exist very long without them. It is no longer wise to view these microbes as something that we can live without. Many scientists now refer to them as crucial. Some refer to the collective 100 trillion microbes (microbiome) as an organ that is as important as the brain or liver.

The tide has indeed turned and we now seek to know as much as we can about our microbial companions. In the ten-year period from 2004 to 2014, the study of the human microbiome has undergone amazing growth. With 160 studies in 2004 to over 3,700 studies in 2014, interest in this area of science doesn't appear to be slowing down anytime soon.

Scientists are coming together to find out more about this pivotal part of the body. The Human Microbiome Project and the American Gut Project are making giant strides forward in the understanding about this internal ecosystem.

ALERT

The American Gut Project allows you to get involved and submit your own samples to find out more about the composition of your intestinal flora and how it may be affecting your life. For $99, you can learn more about your gut microbiome's unique fingerprint. Go to *http://humanfoodproject.com/americangut*.

We are still early on in our understanding of the importance of the microbiome, but so far we know that these microbes encase us in a protective bubble that helps us digest foods, synthesize vitamins and nutrients, regulate immune function, transform chemicals, heavy metals, and radiation, influence brain function and growth, sustain pregnancies, and much more. With the ability to influence our thinking and behavior, some scientists are wondering if perhaps we are mere puppets for the advancement of the microbiome. What has become apparent is that we are so interconnected with them that their health equals our health. How we treat them determines how healthy we will be.

Diet

It has been said that you are what you eat, and some people have taken that statement further and stated that you are what you absorb from what you eat. In both cases, what you eat seems to be a key role in your nutrition status, health, and ability to rebound from various conditions that can affect the body. As you learn more about the gut microbiome, you also learn more about what to feed yourself and maybe more importantly, what to feed them. What you eat can change the composition of the gut almost instantly, for the better or for the worse, so you need to be constantly mindful of how your diet can affect you.

The Good-Old Days

It wasn't so long ago that whole foods that were raised locally by farmers, or in our own backyards, made up the lion's share of our diets. We were very much aware of how our food choices would determine if we were going to be healthy or sick. With industrialization, however, we have ventured farther and farther away from the diet of our grandparents. Now, in the age of the microbiome, we our rediscovering our dietary roots and gaining valuable insights into the benefits of whole foods.

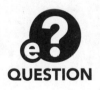

QUESTION

What foods are most important for a healthy lifestyle?
In the Blue Zones study by National Geographic and longevity researchers in 2004, it was found that the diet of many people who lived to the age of 100 and older was predominantly 80 percent plant-based. Meat consumption was about five times per month.

Unlike many processed foods, whole foods are anti-inflammatory in most instances. They are naturally loaded with vitamins, minerals, phytochemicals, fiber, and other nutrients that provide the body with the essential tools necessary for health. Organic whole foods that are free of chemicals should always be your first choice whenever possible. Eating minimally processed foods means that more enzymes and nutrients will be available to you, as food processing can deplete whole foods of these vital factors.

The American Gut Project is another resource that is helping to highlight the importance of plants in the diet as well as a wide variety of them. Fiber, especially the resistant starch type that is a food for the bacteria of the large intestine, as opposed to the small intestine, appears to be very important for a healthy microbiome, and therefore a healthy gut and body.

A SAD Way to Live

How appropriate is it that the acronym for the Standard American Diet spells SAD? Anywhere that this diet is introduced in the world results in an increase in metabolic diseases such as hypertension, diabetes, obesity, and cardiovascular disease, just to name a few. Also known as the Western Diet, this standard way of eating leads to runaway levels of inflammation, nutritional deficiencies, and an increase in doctor and hospital visits. Anyone who chases the American dream via this way of eating is also chasing the American nightmare.

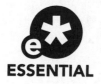

ESSENTIAL

A Western diet is commonly associated with the development of the metabolic syndrome triad of obesity, insulin resistance, and heart disease, with prevalence as high as 84 percent in some countries. The good news is that it is reversible with dietary and lifestyle interventions.

This type of diet is rich in sugar, salt, processed, and fast foods. It's a diet of convenience and the quickest way to join the ranks of the obese, depressed, and medicated.

Gluten-Free

Gluten, a protein found in wheat, barley, and rye, has been found to be very pro-inflammatory. For an increasing number of people, its presence triggers immune system responses that can lead to damage and inflammation in the intestinal tract common to autoimmune celiac disease. Other conditions from asthma to multiple sclerosis have also been linked to gluten in the diet.

While wheat has been a staple of the diet for most every human on the planet for hundreds and thousands of years, its consumption in the United States has fallen due to an increasing percentage of people who are sensitive to gluten. The rise in gluten sensitivity has been attributed to genetically engineered crops, overuse of gluten, and the introduction of antibiotics in the late 1940s and early 1950s. There is no solid consensus on the cause of increased gluten sensitivity.

Interestingly, if we look closely, we find that a protein found in the cell wall of candida, hyphal cell wall protein (HWP-1), is exactly identical to the gliadin proteins that combine to form gluten. This is a classic example of how substances that mirror other substances in the body lead to autoimmune conditions. From this data, it seems likely that correcting fungal candida imbalances in the body may also correct gluten sensitivity issues.

Lifestyle

Lifestyle is another area that can affect gut health. Stress and tension can impact the function of the digestive tract via the vagus nerve. The vagus nerve innervates the small intestine, large intestine, stomach, liver, and pancreas, as well as the brain, heart, and lungs. Depression and anxiety also impact digestive function via the vagus nerve. Many pathways in the body are a two-way street. Digestive imbalances can impact the nervous system function and play a role in stress-related conditions, as well as ADD, ADHD, autism, depression, anxiety, headaches, and many more. As mentioned previously, diet is a big factor in health.

FACT

The vagus nerve, also known as the wanderer, is the longest cranial nerve, originating in the cranium and traveling all the way down to the rectum. It is a major pathway between the gut's brain, the enteric nervous system (ENS), and the head's brain, the central nervous system (CNS).

Meditation, prayer, tai chi, yoga, and exercise can positively impact gut health by countering stressful lifestyle factors. As it seems with almost everything else, finding a place of balance can offset the negative effects of so many aspects of life. The gut can be a key factor in health and disease, depending on how this ecosystem is maintained. While antibiotics can save lives, they have a devastating effect on gut health and can affect everything else in the body. Normal microbes can become pathogenic nightmares, unless we are good stewards of this ecosystem.

CHAPTER 7

Natural Solutions

The natural approach to addressing autoimmune conditions is the foundation of many successful treatment plans. Using science-based evidence and centuries of clinical experience, the holistic doctor and the integrative medical practitioner have the upper hand and offer the best hope for recovery from many autoimmune conditions. This is exciting news for patients and healthcare practitioners alike, as an autoimmune diagnosis no longer has to mean a life sentence of disease and discomfort, as it did in the past.

Vitamins

Perhaps at no other time in history is the use of vitamins as great as it is today. Billions of dollars are spent each year on supplements, as millions of people everywhere look for safe and effective ways to prevent and cure diseases. Following closely behind the success of the clinical and personal use of supplements, science is building a body of evidence that validates the long history of their use in healthcare.

Over 150 million Americans take supplements on a daily basis for prevention and treatment of diseases. Some follow the recommended daily allowance (RDA) as set forth by the Institute of Medicine. The RDA was established over seventy years ago and only considers what a healthy person might need as a daily nutritional requirement. Others choose to take higher amounts due to the constant criticism of the RDA as being too low for anyone dealing with a disease or health condition. Many holistic doctors use much higher, or therapeutic, dosages to treat their patients. Researchers from Norway found that 20–50 percent of hospitalized patients were malnourished.

ALERT

Vitamins and minerals might interact with medications, so it is best to consult with a doctor before taking them together. In general, vitamins and minerals are safe with medications, but they may interfere with some medications and reduce their effectiveness.

In treating autoimmune conditions, the choice of supplements varies from all-purpose multivitamins to specific nutrients related to various conditions. In all instances, a holistic practitioner will recommend that you obtain as many of your nutrients from foods as possible and use supplements to fill in any gaps or additional needs.

Multivitamin and Mineral

Multivitamin and mineral formulas are primarily designed to fill in gaps when the daily requirement of nutrients is not being met by a person's diet. At times when diet is adequate but excess stress and health challenges are present, additional amounts may be necessary. Many people are suffering from what is being called a silent epidemic of hidden hunger, whereby a chronic lack of essential nutrients is contributing to increased levels of sickness and disease in over 2 billion people worldwide, yearly. A 2012 Canadian study showed that multivitamins were able to reduce tissue changes caused by chemicals. Bruce Ames, PhD, a recipient of the National Medal of Science and professor emeritus of biochemistry and molecular biology, University of California, Berkeley, states that vitamins can prevent DNA changes that lead to cancer and other diseases.

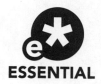

ESSENTIAL

Nutritional needs vary from person to person, day to day, and condition to condition. Young children and the elderly may require more or less of certain nutrients depending on their body's needs and requirements. Pregnant women tend to need more of many nutrients to help support the baby's growth and needs. Most people with any type of sickness require more nutrients to support detoxification and repair.

Dr. Ames's findings are consistent with findings in the Physicians' Health Study at Harvard Medical School, which showed that "taking a standard multivitamin-mineral pill every day for more than a decade reduces the odds of developing cancer."

Autoimmune diseases during pregnancy increase the risk of preterm deliveries and low birth weight. A 2014 study by Johns Hopkins Bloomberg School of Public Health researchers found that taking a multivitamin and mineral formula had a significant impact on increasing low birth weight and decreasing preterm deliveries. The researchers believe that the results were due to the nutritional effect of the multivitamin-mineral on the immune system and inflammation.

Multivitamins are more convenient than carrying around twenty-five bottles of single nutrients, but overall they contain smaller amounts of specific nutrients that someone might need to successfully treat certain conditions. In those instances taking individual nutrients in addition to the multivitamin-mineral can be helpful.

Vitamin C

Vitamin C is a common component of many people's daily arsenal for maintaining health. Vitamin C is commonly supplied as ascorbic acid, but it may come in more natural forms like rose hips, or buffered forms that combine it with calcium, potassium, magnesium, or sodium salts to reduce its acidity. Vitamin C has long been recognized for its ability to stimulate immune system function, as well as its function in tissue repair and protection. It is a strong antioxidant that can help modulate immune system function and reduce inflammation.

FACT

High amounts of vitamin C are stored in the adrenals, the stress gland of the body. Stress depletes the adrenals of vitamin C and vitamin C deficiency further stresses the adrenals. Combat stress and autoimmune diseases by consuming vitamin C daily.

Most doctors recommend amounts that are much higher than the daily RDA of a meager 75–90 mg. High-dose vitamin C of 5,000–20,000 mg has been used successfully by MDs like Frederick Klenner for many decades. Researchers in Japan found that its use was able to "help control autoimmune disease and allergy."

Vitamin D

If there is one vitamin that everyone facing some type of autoimmune challenge should take, it is vitamin D, the king of inflammatory and autoimmune treatments. Vitamin D, technically a hormone, is known to cause many diseases when it is deficient and to cure many more when it is used as a part of a healing therapy. For decades, the RDA for vitamin D (200–400 IU) has been so small that vitamin D's true potential has been hidden. Newer recommendations for daily intake fluctuate from 1,000 to 2,000 IUs, with many people taking even greater amounts. It's not uncommon to hear of doctors starting patients off on amounts of 2,000 IUs or more.

Can someone take too much vitamin D?
The Institute of Medicine states that taking more than the upper limit of 10,000 IU daily of vitamin D may have some risks. Other sources cite that 10,000 IU daily is safe and some doctors recommend as much as 50,000 IU daily for some conditions. Check with your doctor to be sure.

Oxford University genetic researcher Sreeram Ramagopalan states that "genes involved in autoimmune disease and cancer were regulated by vitamin D." He recommends at least 1,000–2,000 IU of vitamin D daily, but cites a Harvard University study in which a dosage of 4,000 IU daily was safe and useful in preventing multiple sclerosis.

Researchers from all over the world continually site the importance of taking vitamin D to treat, reduce, and prevent autoimmune diseases. The benefits of vitamin D have been found to increase with the dosage, creating what researchers identify as a dose-response effect.

The benefits of vitamin D supplementation have been found to extend to cancers, infectious diseases, and other health concerns. While there are no magic pills, vitamin D supplements may be the closest that science has been able to come to providing one.

Vitamin E

Vitamin E, once known as the fertility vitamin for its beneficial effects in helping to establish pregnancies, is also known for its great antioxidant qualities and its ability to protect the nervous system.

ALERT

Vitamin E can have a thinning effect on the blood and its use in combination with blood-thinning medications should be assessed carefully. This usually occurs at high doses and shouldn't be a risk at smaller doses that follow the recommended daily allowance.

Vitamin E is a fat-soluble vitamin that works well with other fats. Vitamin E in combination with fish oils was found to "delay the progress of certain autoimmune diseases" and "decrease levels of pro-inflammatory chemokines" by researchers from the State University of New York.

When choosing a good source of vitamin E, look for the natural tocopherol and tocotrienols forms, as most sources recommend against using the synthetic (dl-) form. The presence of inflammation and autoimmune conditions is an indication that the normal daily maintenance dose of 22 IUs is probably not sufficient. The Institute of Medicine has established 1,500 IUs as the upper tolerable limit of vitamin E intake, although another study showed that 5,500 IUs per day was safe. Consult with a professional to determine which dosage amount works best.

Vitamin A/Beta-Carotene

Vitamin A has long been known for its ability to enhance immune function. Equally as well known is its inactive precursor form, beta-carotene, one of the group of carotenoid pigments that give plants their colors.

FACT

Animal foods contain vitamin A in its preformed state, while plants contain vitamin A as carotenoids, a provitamin A form that is converted to active vitamin A in the body. The most common carotenoid provitamin A forms are alpha-carotene, beta-carotene, and beta-cryptoxanthin. Lutein, zeaxanthin, and lycopene are other common carotenoids, but they have no vitamin A activity.

Vitamin A deficiency has been associated with autoimmune diseases such a lupus, type 1 diabetes, and rheumatoid arthritis. Researchers at Emory University's Woodruff Health Sciences Center found that vitamin A was responsible for calming down immune system responses associated with autoimmune responses. Deficiencies of vitamin A would explain the runaway inflammation associated with autoimmune diseases.

Vitamin A is also known for its ability to negate the production of pro-inflammatory Th17 cells and modulate the activation of pro- and anti-inflammatory immune responses. Combining vitamins A, C, and E along with a multivitamin-mineral formula can enhance the protective and antioxidant effect of each. The synergistic effect was found to have significance in a 2010 study by researchers at Harvard School of Public Health.

The upper limit of vitamin A intake is 10,000 IU per day and going over this amount can be toxic. Beta-carotene, the precursor form, can be taken in much greater amounts. This allows the body to convert as much of the beta-carotene as needed to the active vitamin A form. Using beta-carotene allows the body's wisdom to take the lead to greater health.

B Vitamins

B vitamins play a role in so many functions of the body that ensuring optimal levels of these vitamins is one of the best ways to address vitamin deficiencies that can cause havoc in cases of autoimmunity.

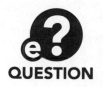

QUESTION

Why do B vitamins turn the urine yellow?
Other than B_6, it's difficult to absorb too much of a B vitamin, as elevated levels in the blood cause active excretion of B vitamins in the urine due to their water solubility. Taking a B vitamin complex can help ensure proper absorption of all B vitamins.

Humans need B vitamins from their diet, as the body does not store B vitamins. Microbes in the intestinal tract can also produce these vitamins, however. The presence or absence of B vitamins can signal immune responses that increase or decrease inflammation as evidenced by a group of Australian researchers. Imbalances within the gut are common with autoimmune diseases and can signal an imbalance in the production of B vitamins by gut microflora as well.

Vitamin B_1

Vitamin B_1, or thiamine, plays a role in the metabolism of carbohydrates for healthy brain and nervous system function, as well as for other tissues. Italian researchers found that as a treatment therapy in autoimmune thyroiditis, thiamine "led to a partial or complete regression of the fatigue and related disorders" of patients. The recommended daily dose for adults is 1.2 mg per day.

Vitamin B$_2$

Vitamin B$_2$ (riboflavin) helps convert carbohydrates into energy, and it also exhibits antioxidant functions that can help reduce inflammation. Riboflavin may also play a role in reducing fatigue in autoimmune conditions. Taking 1.6 mg per day is the recommended amount, although higher doses have been used.

Vitamin B$_3$

Vitamin B$_3$ (niacin) is required for over 400 enzymes used in vital reactions in the body. A deficiency of niacin could lead to imbalances that create inflammation, autoimmune diseases, advanced aging, and cancers.

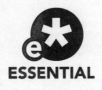

ESSENTIAL

Niacin often causes a flushing response that can last for 1–2 hours. To avoid this, you can take slow-release forms of niacin, such as inositol nicotinate, inositol hexanicotinate, or niacinamide. Niacin is the only form of vitamin B$_3$ that has been shown in studies to lower cholesterol, as evidenced by researchers from Harvard and Beth Israel Deaconess Medical Center in Boston, Massachusetts.

The recommended dosage is 30 mg per day. Some studies report dosages as high as 2,000–3,000 mg per day are necessary in order to lower blood lipid levels. Niacin can cause a flushing response that turns the skin a reddish color temporarily.

Vitamin B$_6$

Vitamin B$_6$ (pyridoxine) is an important B vitamin that together with vitamins B$_{12}$ and B$_9$ (folic acid) form a B vitamin triad that helps each of these three B vitamins to function more effectively. Taking B$_6$ along with B$_{12}$ and folic acid can reduce inflammation in the body. Low levels of B$_6$ are associated with rheumatoid arthritis, celiac disease, Crohn's disease, ulcerative colitis, and inflammatory bowel disease. B$_6$ deficiency also can lower the clearance of estrogen and decrease white blood cell production, both of which affect autoimmune responses.

The daily requirement for most adults is around 1.3 mg.

Vitamin B$_{12}$

Vitamin B$_{12}$ (cobalamin) is an important B vitamin with a complex structure that enables it to play a role in many areas of health for the body. Unlike other B vitamins, B$_{12}$ is stored in the body and primarily in the liver. It is important for the absorption of folic acid, neurological and cardiovascular function, red blood cell formation, and the synthesis of DNA, the cells' building blocks.

ALERT

Vitamin B$_{12}$, like many other vitamins, has a tendency to be deficient in the elderly due to decreased absorption and changes in the levels of hydrochloric acid in the stomach and bacterial flora in the intestinal tract. Increased dosages are often necessary to meet their daily requirements.

Like vitamin E and vitamin D, vitamin B$_{12}$ deficiency is often considered a silent epidemic in the United States. Deficiencies can lead to anemia and increased levels of inflammation that affect several systems in the body. The daily recommended amount in the United States is 2.4 mcg per day, while elsewhere in the world it can be much higher. A study by researchers in Japan found that massive doses of B$_{12}$ daily (60 mg, 25,000 times the U.S. RDA) was able to improve certain markers in multiple sclerosis. Red meats are a good source of B$_{12}$, which is why many vegetarians and vegans are deficient in B$_{12}$.

Folic Acid

Folic acid (vitamin B$_9$, or folate) is an essential nutrient that most foods are fortified with, making deficiencies unlikely. Due to its link with neural tube and congenital defects in newborn babies, folic acid fortification was begun in 1996 in the United States and other countries.

FACT

The Centers for Disease Control recommends that women who intend to get pregnant start taking folic acid for at least a month before getting pregnant. This often means that women who are fertile and open to getting pregnant should start consuming folic acid, as pregnancies can be unexpected and unplanned in many instances.

Recent discoveries in science have shown that some people are deficient in the enzyme (MTHFR) necessary for the body to process the form of folinic acid used in food fortification. People with a deficiency of this enzyme can use folic acid or methyltetrahydrofolate supplements.

Low folate levels are associated with increased levels of inflammation, cancers, cardiovascular disease, genetic defects, and anemia. The daily recommended amount is 400 mcg. Together with vitamin B_{12}, folic acid helps prevent and assist with many conditions.

Alpha Lipoic Acid

Alpha lipoic acid (ALA) is a powerful antioxidant found in all cells. It is both fat- and water-soluble, allowing it to affect many tissues in the body. It has been found to help balance blood sugar and improve brain function.

With its ability to pass readily into the brain, it can exert a neuroprotective effect that has been found beneficial in multiple sclerosis. Researchers from the National Cancer Research Institute of Genoa, Italy, found that ALA suppressed inflammatory Th1 and Th2 cytokines and was effective at interfering with the autoimmune reaction.

The recommended dosage varies between 50–600 mg daily depending on the source, as there is no RDA for this nutrient. Some studies have used dosages as high as 1,800 mg per day.

Fish Oils

Fish oils are high in omega-3 polyunsaturated fatty acids, which have been found to reduce inflammation and autoimmune diseases in a number of clinical studies, where they have demonstrated significant benefits. The two main fatty acid components in fish oil are eicosapentaenoic acid (EPA) and docosahexaenoic acid (DHA).

Cod liver oil is an excellent example of a beneficial fish oil. Cod liver oil, which contains EPA, DHA, and vitamins A and D, has been used for centuries to treat inflammation, rheumatoid arthritis, and a number of other diseases and conditions. Some earlier practices even called for the cod livers to ferment naturally in the open air before extraction of the oils. Natural manufacturing practices have eliminated the bad taste that was associated with cod liver oil until the late twentieth century.

ALERT

Large fish with high amounts of fat and therefore omega-3 fatty acids may also contain higher levels of fat-soluble toxins. Examples of this are shark, swordfish, tuna, and tilefish, which can contain high levels of mercury and other toxins. Eating fewer of these types of fish is seen as a safe dietary practice.

Minerals

The benefits of minerals in treating autoimmune disorders are less known than those of vitamins. This may be more due to the fact that most doctors aren't as well educated about minerals as they are about vitamins. To a certain degree, it can also reflect the complexity of how minerals interact with other nutrients to create the positive effect associated with them. This is often seen in the interaction between certain minerals and their vitamin counterparts.

Calcium

Calcium deficiency has been found to play a role in many conditions and usually includes a simultaneous deficiency of vitamin D. Since vitamin D affects calcium directly, this relationship is very understandable. Any vitamin D deficiency can also create a calcium deficiency and all the diseases and conditions that go with it. Among the conditions representing both nutrients are cardiovascular diseases, cancers, type 1 diabetes, irritable bowel syndrome, metabolic syndrome, and osteoporosis.

ESSENTIAL

The various types of calcium formulas on the market have different absorption rates. Calcium carbonate has the lowest absorption rate, while calcium citrate and malate forms have higher absorption rates. The highest rate of absorption is associated with calcium bisglycinate. In all instances, at least twice the RDA may be necessary to meet nutritional needs.

The RDA for calcium is 1,000 mg in adults, and increases to 1,200 mg a day in women older than fifty. A German study in 2010 found that only 32 percent of Americans and 50 percent of Germans met their daily requirement of calcium.

Magnesium

Magnesium deficiencies often go together with calcium deficiencies. Magnesium is a cofactor in hundreds of reactions in the body and deficiencies can have a wide impact on health and disease. Magnesium absorption is dependent on a healthy digestive tract. Deficiencies are associated with autoimmune thyroid, intestinal inflammation, cardiovascular disease, and diabetes.

The recommended dosage ranges from 400 to 420 mg per day in adult males. In women, the RDA ranges from 310 to 360 mg a day. Taking too much magnesium is unlikely, although it may cause diarrhea.

Zinc

Zinc is one of the primary minerals of the immune system. Like calcium and magnesium, zinc requires an intact digestive tract for best absorption. Deficiencies of zinc are associated with multiple conditions, including diabetes, cardiovascular disease, cancer, and autoimmune diseases. The recommended daily intake is 11 mg. Taking over 40 mg of zinc can deplete other essential minerals, like iron and copper.

Selenium

Selenium is a mineral that is often linked with vitamin E for best outcomes. Taking vitamin E and selenium together can provide more benefits than when taking them alone. Selenium deficiency has been linked to autoimmune thyroiditis and Hashimoto's disease by researchers from Germany and the Netherlands. Selenium is thought to play a role in inhibiting thyroid antibodies.

The daily recommended intake is 200 mcg daily. Therapeutic doses may be as high as 400 or 800 mcg daily.

Iodine

Iodine is a trace mineral that also has widespread deficiencies in many people. Like folic acid, fortification of foods was seen as a way to address this widespread deficiency. Iodized table salt is the leading source of iodine for most people. With salt getting more and more bad press, iodine deficiency is seeing a new resurgence. The primary tissue affected by iodine deficiency or excess is the thyroid gland.

QUESTION

What foods are high in iodine?
Generally, seafood has a higher amount of iodine than other foods. Seaweed and kelp are two good sources of iodine. Eggs and dairy are two other sources of iodine. Himalayan salts are a better source of iodine than regular table salt. Himalayan salts have higher levels of naturally occurring iodine, along with a variety of minerals to support tissue health. Table salt is a processed salt that only provides sodium chloride, along with added iodine and some anti-caking agents to make it flow better.

Studies demonstrate that excess iodine is associated with autoimmune thyroid disease. Others state that iodine is not the problem, but the simultaneous deficiency of magnesium, selenium, and fluoride exposure is creating the negative effects associated with iodine. Working with a doctor is the best way to decide how best to utilize iodine, if at all.

Herbs

The use of herbs has been around for thousands of years. Each country has its own pharmacy of local herbs that have been used for various ailments and diseases. Although it's impossible to consider every herb, a few of the more popular ones can be addressed here.

Andrographis

Andrographis paniculata is an annual herb native to Asia. It is known for its ability to suppress both humoral and cellular immune responses. Its effectiveness has resulted in the development of the drug andrographolide.

In 2009, researchers from Chile showed that andrographis demonstrated a significant effect against rheumatoid arthritis by improving several inflammatory markers of the disease. Patients saw improvement in as little as two weeks by taking extracts three times a day.

Boswellia

Boswellia serrata, commonly known as frankincense, is a tree found in India, Africa, and the Middle East. It has a long history of use against chronic inflammation and pain. Fatty acids found in frankincense have been found to have inhibitory effects against pro-inflammatory immune cells, antibodies, enzymes, and free radicals. This broad range of activity makes it an excellent choice in combatting the chronic inflammation of autoimmune diseases.

FACT

The use of frankincense dates back thousands of years and once was considered a priceless commodity. Egyptians, Greeks, and Romans had many uses for it in addition to its healing properties. Today, scientists are rediscovering the amazing properties of frankincense and its effectiveness in many conditions.

Researchers from India, using the gold standard of testing (randomized, double-blind, placebo-controlled), found frankincense to have safe and tolerable effects in the body. It is considered to be a very strong pain killer and has shown efficacy against the arthritic pain of autoimmune rheumatoid arthritis.

Ginger

Ginger (*Zingiber officinale*) is a well-known herb and spice that has been used for centuries to reduce inflammation. The strong activity of its protease enzymes helps reduce inflammation in a number of autoimmune diseases and makes it a useful substance in any anticancer protocol.

Ginger has historically been used as a cure for several diseases in traditional medicine. Science continues to discover its ability to inhibit some of the body's strongest pro-inflammatory cytokines.

Ginseng

Ginseng is another of the ancient remedies whose effectiveness as a healing agent is still being discovered by many people. Used for thousands of years, the American and Asian forms (*Panax quinquefolius* and *Panax ginseng*) of ginseng are the varieties sought out for their anti-inflammatory properties when treating rheumatoid arthritis, cancer, stress, diabetes, neurodegenerative disorders, and even the common cold.

ALERT

Ginseng can interact with several medications such as ACE inhibitors, MAOIs, blood thinners, diabetic medications, morphine, Lasix, and others. It can also increase the stimulant action of some drugs, including caffeine. Talk with your doctor if you have questions about its use.

The dose-response effect of many herbs applies to ginseng as well, where small dosages may boost certain immune responses and larger ones will suppress them. The dosage is often determined by the condition being treated.

Rosemary

Rosemary is another well-known spice and herb with a history of use as a healing agent. Much of its healing potential is attributed to the rosmarinic acid it contains. It has been used to suppress inflammation in autoimmune conditions like arthritis, thyroiditis, and multiple sclerosis. Whether used as a way to add flavor to meals or as a healing agent, rosemary can have a significant effect when used on a frequent basis.

Turmeric

Turmeric (also known as curcumin) is the number one reigning anti-inflammatory spice at the moment. Turmeric has a long, colorful history dating back over 4,000 years. Science's love affair with this golden spice has generated over 3,000 publications over the past thirty years citing the importance of turmeric. Turmeric has been an important part of ancient Ayurvedic and Chinese medicines, and now modern medicine. Its potent anti-inflammatory, antioxidant, antimicrobial, antiseptic, and anticancer properties make it an essential part of hundreds of treatments. Its effectiveness against depression and stress make it an important part of any mind-body approach to healing.

ESSENTIAL

Turmeric comes from the ginger family of plants and resembles ginger closely. Its usefulness in treating a wide variety of conditions is reflected in the ancient Sanskrit language, in which it has fifty-three different names.

Beyond its almost miraculous effectiveness, turmeric is also considered very safe, with no history of toxicity associated with its use. It is also a very cost-effective choice for the masses in this era of high-priced medical care. Anyone who is serious about her health will be serious about using turmeric on a daily basis.

Changshan

This relative newcomer on the list of herbal healing agents only has a 2,000-year-old history as a healing agent. Scientists at the Harvard School of Dental Medicine have found that components of changshan are responsible for suppressing the pro-inflammatory actions of the Th17 immune cells found in many autoimmune conditions. This type of effect makes changshan an effective choice for conditions such as psoriasis, rheumatoid arthritis, multiple sclerosis, and inflammatory bowel disease.

Getting Healthy with Dirt: The Hygiene Hypothesis

The hygiene hypothesis suggests that an excessively clean environment alters normal development of the immune system and its ability to tolerate a world filled with microbes. This loss of immune tolerance leads to excessive and chronic levels of inflammation that can play a role in asthma, allergies, and autoimmune diseases. Today's lifestyles continually remove us farther and farther from the natural environment and enshroud us in an antiseptic, antimicrobial world where the immune system is uneducated, and therefore unprepared to handle anything but a sterile environment.

Scientists point out that once-rare allergic and autoimmune conditions have now become "epidemic" in our modern world. Infectious diseases are more rampant than ever before, in spite of our efforts to eradicate them with antibiotics and other antimicrobials.

Conversely, in countries where exposure to nature, dirt, and microbes remains high, the occurrence of allergies and autoimmune diseases remains very low.

Worm Therapy

The use of worms in therapy is attracting more and more attention. University of Iowa researcher Joel Weinstock used noninfectious helminth worms in patients with Crohn's disease and ulcerative colitis and achieved a success rate of almost 80 percent. Researchers in other countries have obtained similar results. Dr. Weinstock points out that "90 percent of Venezuelan Indians living in the rainforest had worms and no allergies. Of the more affluent Venezuelans living in the cities, only 10 percent had light worm infections and 43 percent had allergies."

FACT

The use of helminth worms as a therapy is not yet FDA approved in the United States, forcing some businesses to set up shop just across the border in Tijuana, Mexico. The therapy can include swallowing 2,500 microscopic parasite eggs every three weeks for the duration of the treatment period.

The use of worms may have other implications in the treatment of a number of autoimmune diseases like multiple sclerosis that are increasingly linked to the health of the gut.

Fecal Transplants

Fecal transplants, or fecal bacteriotherapy, in which the feces of one person is taken and implanted into another person, has shown tremendous benefits in some instances. Life-threatening diarrhea is one example where the use of fecal transplants was able to create a 90 percent cure rate. The common approach used in administering fecal transplants is either via enemas or colonoscopy implants. In the past, donors have typically been family members, but newer stringent screening methods are enabling qualified donors to contribute as well.

While the appeal of what is being called poo therapy is understandably low, its success rate is something that the use of medicines is unable to come close to. Given the choice between worm therapy and fecal therapy, it may be that playing in the dirt more often will be the easiest and most appealing way to address the problems of an overly hygienic world. Allowing nature to play a greater role in our lives can enable us to have a healthier and longer life.

CHAPTER 8

The Autoimmune Diet

As much as diets are based on the preferences that any one individual, group, or culture chooses to follow at any given time, the autoimmune diet is something different in that many people must follow it for health reasons. As time marches on, however, it is likely that almost everyone will need to follow the autoimmune diet periodically, or even permanently if they hope to maintain a healthy life. While following this type of diet is becoming less of a preference and more of a necessity, it doesn't have to be a challenge or feel like a jail sentence. With the right approach, it can lead to a life of liberation!

Cooling the Fires with Gluten-Free Foods

If there's anything that science excels at in the area of autoimmune diseases and related discoveries, it is its ability to help define the triggers that are associated with autoimmune diseases. While there is probably still enough mystery to keep scientists busy for generations to come, there is now a clearer picture of what you can eat, and what you should avoid eating, in order to stay healthy and get healthy.

One of the clearest examples of this are the scientific discoveries of the influence of gluten on inflammation and autoimmunity. Gluten has been associated with conditions like celiac disease and non-celiac gluten sensitivity in which its presence in foods and food-like substances has a major impact on the health of the digestive tract. It has also been associated with diseases that are more remote to the digestive tract, such as arthritis, multiple sclerosis, schizophrenia, and asthma.

The public concern over the impact of gluten-laden foods now exceeds the number of people who are diagnosed with celiac disease. While only around 1 percent of the population is diagnosed with the most severe form of gluten intolerance known as celiac disease, according to David Perlmutter, MD, author of *Grain Brain*, it may be affecting over 40 percent of the population. At any rate, concern over gluten-containing foods is driving gluten-free food sales in the billions of dollars.

Given that gluten has been associated with driving autoimmune diseases and inflammation, and inflammation is associated with almost every disease, it makes sense that avoiding gluten can help cool the fires that drive autoimmunity and other diseases.

How the Autoimmune Diet Works

The goal of the autoimmune diet is to not only avoid exposures to substances that can fuel and drive inflammation and therefore autoimmunity, but also to supply the body with foods and nutrients that promote and drive health. By following a few simple practices, you can make a substantial difference in your quality of life.

Organic

Organic foods have many advantages, especially if they are whole foods. They provide vitamins, minerals, antioxidants, and the necessary building blocks that create a healthy body. A 2002 study by Italian researchers found higher antioxidant levels in organic foods, and a 2014 study by researchers from the United Kingdom found that "concentrations of a range of antioxidants such as polyphenolics were found to be substantially higher," in the range of 19–69 percent higher.

ALERT

Organic does not mean completely chemical-free. Pesticides with some degree of toxicity that are approved for use on organic foods include rotenone, pyrethrin, and spinosad. Copper, a natural substance, is often used and may present problems when large amounts are present on foods over time.

Organic foods are also free of the antibiotics that are used in conventional food practices. Researchers from Mayo Clinic have noted a four-fold increase in the incidence of celiac disease since 1950, a time period that coincides with the introduction of antibiotics and the proliferation of fungal candida growth in humans. Candida contains a hyphal cell wall protein (HWP1) that is identical to the gliadin proteins that make up gluten. HWP1 is a transglutaminase enzyme and human antibodies to transglutaminase are the hallmark of celiac disease.

Chemicals

Over 10,000 chemicals are allowed for direct use in food processing, and over 650,000 other chemicals present in the environment can find their way into foods. By avoiding hundreds of thousands of chemicals, the incidence of inflammation and disease-promoting factors is greatly reduced. Environmental exposure to chemicals is consistently cited as a cause of autoimmunity. A 1988 study at the University of Connecticut stated that "autoimmune responses and/or autoimmune diseases are induced in humans and experimental animals by chronic exposure to various chemicals." A common form of chemicals that few people consider are medication residues. The U.S. Geological Survey states that "nearly 80 percent of rivers tested contained traces of residues" and a 2002 University of Cincinnati College of Medicine study cited the "relationship of certain medications to lupus and other auto-immune conditions" with over seventy such medications related to autoimmune diseases.

GMOs

Are genetically modified foods (GMOs) a threat? Science seems to be split on this issue, with more scientists opposing the threat than those that support it. Many developed nations on the other hand do not consider GMOs to be safe and have banned or severely restricted them.

QUESTION

Have GMOs been proven to harm humans?
There are several studies that look at the effects of GMOs on humans and animals and none are without criticisms from other scientists. This is a hotly contested area that polarizes people on both sides. Labeling products to allow people to make their own choice may be the best middle ground until the science is all in.

Currently, the threat to the environment appears to be more substantiated than the threat to humans, but that can change quickly as science learns more. A growing consumer-driven movement against GMOs is creating greater degrees of transparency in the manufacturing and marketing of foods, which allows consumers to know more about what's in their foods. This could eventually lead to greater recognition of the relationship between foods and autoimmune disease.

People who are interested in avoiding GMO foods can look for the Non-GMO Project label on foods and drinks. This detailed assessment of foods traces the ingredients all the way back to their origin to help ensure that no GMOs were used in bringing those foods to market. The stringent verification program used by the Non-GMO Project is daunting to say the least, and not without its critics.

Common Allergens

Science has identified a group of allergens that many people are already having problems with. The list of eight common allergens as found on most labels includes wheat, soy, dairy, peanuts, shellfish, fish, eggs, and tree nuts. Unfortunately, other foods are appearing on labels here and there, and the list is likely to continue growing. Corn, yeast, sesame, and stone fruits (apricots, peaches, plums, and nectarines) are popping up here and there as additional allergens.

ESSENTIAL

For those who are uncertain as to whether they have any food allergies, they can consult a holistic practitioner and find out more about ways to test for food allergens. Some common ways to check for food allergies are skin prick allergy tests, IgE blood tests, and the ALCAT sensitivity test.

Allergens promote inflammatory responses in the body that can cause flare-ups of existing conditions, or add to the development of others. Avoiding food allergens is a way to put out fires before they begin.

Nature's Answers

Part of the amazing wonder of nature is how, despite man's many mistakes throughout time, nature seems to at least be able to offer solutions to help offset man's short-sided creations. This magnificent design can be seen in the nutrients and antioxidants found in foods, herbs, and spices.

Foods

Fruit and veggies have proven themselves through the trials of time and the strict standards of testing. Their ability to influence the activation or deactivation of genes indicates that they hold a unique position in the outcomes of disease. Not only can they prevent the genes of diseases from being turned on, but they can also silence the genes of disease that have been turned on. From this viewpoint, no disease is permanent and every cure is possible. Fruit and vegetables are best when they are fresh, as nature intended them to be. Cooking and processing them can rob them of nutrients and concentrate sugars.

Spices and Herbs

Spices and herbs, like fruit and veggies, have also demonstrated their abilities to turn on and off human genes. Name a disease and you're likely to find several spices and herbs that have been shown to prevent, cure, or treat it. Turmeric is racking up an impressive resume of scientific studies and clinical trials that prove its superiority to medications in many instances. Other popular healing spices include ginger, sage, rosemary, black cumin, pomegranate, and allspice.

Water

Getting enough water for the body to function properly is often forgotten due to water's constant presence in most people's lives. Dehydration, however, often goes undiagnosed and can result in many health complications and symptoms that may mimic certain autoimmune diseases. Ensuring adequate water intake can help maintain balance and homeostatic function of the body's internal environment.

Foods and juices can supply some of the body's daily water requirements, but any detoxification process may require you to be constantly aware of meeting your body's demands. While there's no set rule on how much water each person needs, anyone dealing with an autoimmune condition, which usually indicates increased levels of inflammation, will have to consider taking more than the minimal daily recommendations.

FACT

Dehydration happens very quickly and often goes unrecognized. It only takes a 1–2 percent loss of the body's water content to create dehydration in an individual. Pregnancy and aging causes higher fluid requirements than normal. Most people are already dehydrated by the time they are thirsty.

The traditional rule on water has been eight (8-ounce) glasses of water a day. Other sources have stated as much as 1 quart for every 50 pounds of body weight. Whatever guidelines you follow, remember to factor in age, weight, weather conditions, activity levels, health conditions, and the use of any medications. Drinking a little more than you think you need might be a good rule to follow.

Make sure that the water has been purified to avoid chemicals that only add to the body's toxic load. Reverse osmosis and carbon block systems are both good ways to purify water. Top of the line systems will include both, with some additional measures thrown in to ensure the purest drinking water available.

Detoxifying Your Meals

An autoimmune diet protocol provides a solid foundation for creating health with every meal. In addition to supplying wholesome foods that nourish, repair, and restore the body, it can also provide foods that enable the body to detoxify and manage the effects of living in a toxic world.

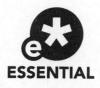

ESSENTIAL

The main detoxification organ of the body is the liver. Helping out the liver are the kidneys, bowels, lungs, and skin. Most detoxification protocols address assisting the liver. As chemicals are removed from the blood by the liver, they can then be bound to fats in the bile to be released through the bowels. Keeping the bowels moving helps improve liver function.

Every meal can be used to take you one or even several steps closer to a healthy mind and body. Each meal can positively modify your genetics and play a role in silencing genes associated with diseases. With fruit and vegetables leading the way, you can eat your way to health by countering the effects of toxins that create disease. As Hippocrates is credited with saying, "Let food be thy medicine."

Apples

Most everyone is familiar with the phrase "An apple a day, keeps the doctor away." It's a statement that is supported by centuries of use and years of research, as apples provide many benefits. In addition to the vitamins, minerals, antioxidants and polyphenols, apples are a good source of fiber, and specifically the soluble pectin fiber that is known to help detoxify heavy metals and chemicals found in foods. Apples are also rich in flavonoids, which are known to suppress cancers and tumor formation, and don't forget about the D-glucarate that helps neutralize toxins. Not bad for a common fruit that many people often pass up for sugary snacks.

Artichokes

Artichokes have a centuries-old reputation for their ability to assist with liver function and detoxification. Artichokes also help stimulate the flow of bile from the gall bladder, which in turn helps to bind toxins. Artichokes aren't as easy to grab and eat as apples, but they can be worth the little effort needed to bring their abilities to the forefront in detoxifying the body.

Avocados

Raw fats can be very beneficial in any detoxification process, making avocados an excellent choice. Avocados are high in glutathione, which supports one of the main detoxification pathways of the body. Like many of the detoxification foods, they assist the liver and can help prevent liver damage caused by toxins. Enjoy them raw as much as possible.

Beets

Beets are a good blood purifier and stimulate liver function. With a high antioxidant profile, as is evidenced by their rich red color, they can have a strong anti-inflammatory effect.

One class of these newly discovered antioxidants are the betalains that Israeli researchers found may "provide protection against certain oxidative disorders in humans." Examples of oxidative disorders are neurodegenerative diseases like Alzheimer's and Parkinson's, and cardiovascular diseases such as hypertension, atherosclerosis, and heart failure.

Don't be surprised if the color of your urine or stool turns red when eating beets. The betanin pigment in beets is responsible for this startling change. The color change is only temporary and should be gone within 48–60 hours.

Broccoli

Broccoli contains a potent nutrient called sulforaphane, which is known for its anti-inflammatory and detoxification boosting powers. Sulforaphanes can help reduce blood pressure and fight prostate, breast, lung, and bladder cancers. Broccoli can be a very important food due to its ability to counter the effects of estrogen and estrogenic chemicals in the body. With women having a higher incidence of autoimmune diseases, broccoli may be a necessary mainstay of the diet.

Cabbage

Cabbage has many of the benefits of broccoli, as it also contains sulforaphanes. Both broccoli and cabbage belong to the family of cruciferous vegetables, and both have excellent antiestrogen effects that can help reduce the risk of many conditions. Cabbage helps support some of the main detoxification pathways of the body that reduce the effect of environmental toxins.

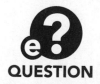

QUESTION

Is it safe to eat cabbage if I have a thyroid problem?
Cabbage, broccoli, cauliflower, Brussels sprouts, kale, collards, and bok choy are all cruciferous vegetables and known goitrogens. Goitrogens can enlarge the thyroid and slow down its function. They accomplish this by interfering with iodine usage and thyroid hormone formation. If you have a slow thyroid, consider eating other vegetables.

Cilantro

Cilantro is an herb that frequently finds it way into many dishes. Also known as coriander, cilantro is an excellent way to detoxify heavy metals that can accumulate in the body. It is more commonly found in Mexican and Asian dishes than American dishes, and its taste tends to make people hate it or love it. The very act of eating cilantro can cause the body to release heavy metals, which may not make someone feel too well, but its regular use can help ensure that harmful levels of heavy metals don't build up in the tissues. As a preventative and a treatment, cilantro is almost a must in today's world.

Celery

Celery is often overlooked when it comes to detoxification and health benefits, but it shouldn't be. It is an excellent source of phytonutrients that can provide anti-inflammatory and antioxidant benefits, and may also provide protection against various cancers and autoimmune diseases. Easy to prepare and easy to carry around without worry of it going bad, celery is an excellent snack that should never be left at home.

Kale

Kale has a history dating back thousands of years. This once popular vegetable fell out of favor, but has recently regained its place in the limelight, and rightfully so. Kale is another of the cruciferous vegetables that impart so many benefits to humans. Its ease of growth makes it an excellent choice for anyone's home garden.

FACT

The cruciferous vegetables were once considered to be the same species of plant. Through cultivation methods and selective propagation, the plants differentiated into the various forms we now consume. The leafy kale plant was much like the present-day cabbage.

Kale is high in vitamins A, C, K, calcium, potassium, and iron. Its anti-inflammatory effect and liver benefits make this leafy vegetable an excellent choice for combatting environmental toxicity.

Lemons and Limes

These two common fruits are almost an afterthought when it comes to beneficial foods, but they both contain powerful nutrients that help reduce the pro-inflammatory effects of many toxins. The high vitamin C content has been shown to protect against many free radicals and autoimmune inflammatory polyarthritis. The contribution of vitamin C to increasing levels of glutathione in the body help ensure that detoxification doesn't get backed up and lead to other imbalances.

Juicing and Cleanses

With many autoimmune conditions, the digestive tract is frequently involved and the ability to digest and absorb foods is often less than optimal. In some instances, juicing can be the best way to supply the necessary nutrients while at the same time delivering them in a liquid form that allows for better absorption and usage. Cleanses, on the other hand, can help release toxins, and in the case of fasts, allow the digestive system a break from constantly having to digest and process foods.

Juicing

Humans lack the necessary enzymes to break down the cellulose walls that are found in many vegetables and fruit. This means that important nutrients are locked away inside cells found in these plants. Animals have the enzymes in their systems to unlock this treasure house of nutrient stores, while cooking and heating processes are necessary for humans to access these nutrients. Unfortunately, many of the nutrients are lost in the cooking process, which makes it a less than optimal choice.

Juicing provides an answer to this dilemma by mechanically breaking down the cellulose walls to release the healing powers contained within plants. This enables many people who have impaired digestive systems the ability to benefit from all that each plant has to offer. Juicing can also be used as a cleanse, or juice fast, which assists with detoxification of the body.

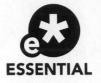

On an anti-inflammatory or autoimmune diet, vegetable juices are a better choice than fruit juices. Mixing a low glycemic fruit such as apples or berries with vegetables is better than using the sweeter fruits like bananas. Avoid juicing only fruits.

The popularity of juicing today means that many people can find a juice store near them if they don't want to go through the expense of having their own juicer. Juice stores typically have industrial strength juicers that effectively break down the cell walls and cellulose to produce juices with high degrees of antioxidant and nutrient activity. Some places even specialize in juice cleanses that are tailored to each individual's needs or to a particular type of cleansing process that addresses the liver or some other tissue in the body.

Cleanses

There are a variety of cleanses available that address a wide range of conditions, from liver/gall bladder cleanses to candida cleanses to whole-body cleanses. Each cleanse will usually have a dietary protocol attached to it, as well as the use of specific foods, juices, or supplements. In many cases, all of these will be used in combination to achieve the best results.

The popularity of candida and heavy metal cleanses means that there are a wide variety of choices available. As cleanses tend to push certain detoxification pathways more than juicing might, working with a holistic practitioner can help make sure that you get the most out the cleansing process in a safe and effective manner.

Focusing on foods, herbs, spices, and supplements that help with detoxification of the liver can be a good way to help reduce inflammation and autoimmune reactions in the body. The higher the toxic load of an individual, the greater the likelihood that she will have inflammation flare-ups.

Juice fasting over short periods of time can be an effective way for some people to jumpstart their body's detoxification process. Detoxification processes in general can require a lot of fuel to run within the body, so strict fasting may work against the process of detoxification in some instances.

Autoimmune Yes and No Foods

There can be great variability in the foods that are acceptable from person to person, but in general, there are certain foods that tend to be more acceptable than others when it comes to autoimmune diets. One way to divide them up is by creating lists of "Yes" and "No" foods, with Yes foods less likely to cause allergic and inflammatory reactions and No foods more likely to do so.

Yes Foods

All Yes foods should be organic as often as possible. Meats should be free-range, grass-fed, wild-caught, hormone-free, and other such labels that reflect conscious farming practices. Oils should be unrefined, virgin oils to avoid high-heat processes that destroy the quality of fatty acids present.

FACT

Most oils undergo a refining process that helps extend their shelf life and stability. Refined vegetable oils tend to have higher levels of the omega-6 oils that are frequently associated with greater levels of inflammation in the body.

Use the following list as a guideline. The variety of sensitivities in today's world means that no one diet fits everyone. Through trial and experience, you will know what works and doesn't work for you. Nightshade vegetables (tomatoes, bell peppers, peppers, potatoes) might not work for some, but might work for others. Coffee may not work for someone with allergies or asthma, but may work for others. Remember that when foods don't work for someone, it may be an indication that the digestive system needs to be repaired. After repairing the gut, many food allergies may disappear. If you have symptoms of gas, bloating, headaches, fatigue, etc., after eating, that can be an indication that a certain food may not work for you at the moment. That's your body's feedback about what works for it and what doesn't. If you have blood sugar regulation issues, low glycemic fruit like berries and apples may work best. Most fruit should be more on the unripe side to avoid excessive sugars—i.e., greenish bananas instead of yellow.

YES FOODS

- All vegetables
- All meats, except pork
- All fresh fruit, except oranges
- Coconut (butter, cream, milk, and water)
- Brown rice, short or long grain
- Brown rice cereal
- Eggs
- Cold-pressed oils (e.g., extra-virgin olive oil, virgin coconut oil)
- Herbs and spices (avoid mixes, which often have fillers)
- Herbal teas
- Apple cider vinegar

No Foods

In general, No foods include everything not mentioned previously. While someone may feel that certain No foods work fine for them, the following ones often create or add to inflammatory reactions and imbalances within the body that may not be immediately felt. The biggest No food in this list is gluten. Becoming familiar with everything that gluten is found in can be accomplished by referencing sites such as *www.gluten.net*, or *www.celiac.org*, as well as books such as *The Everything Guide to Living Gluten Free*. Just because a food is gluten-free doesn't mean it will work on an autoimmune diet. Simple carbs and foods that break down into sugars very quickly can cause blood sugar spikes that drive inflammation. Gluten-free foods plus the Yes foods listed earlier are the better guideline.

One of the biggest ongoing debates is the use of sweeteners other than common sugars. This includes both artificial and natural sweeteners such as stevia. In general, it's best to avoid all of these sweeteners, although natural leaf stevia and raw honey in very small amounts might be the exceptions.

Artificial sweeteners have been linked to an increased risk of diabetes by researchers in Israel, as well as other potential toxicities by researchers from the University of Pennsylvania. Many commercial varieties of stevia are bound to simple sugars, but raw stevia leaf is not. Truly raw honey is always solid at room temperature.

Given the impact of sugars on the body and the development of allergic and conditioned reflexes through exposure, all sweeteners may be problematic. If you're not seeing improvement in your symptoms, exclude all sweeteners, even stevia and raw honey.

NO FOODS
- Gluten—includes condiments, sauces, lunchmeats, sausages, MSG, etc.
- Dairy, including butter, kefir, and cream
- Dried fruit, fruit juice
- Oranges
- Soy products—milk, tempeh, tofu, soy sauce
- Nuts and seeds
- Beans, legumes, and lentils
- All grains except brown rice
- Popcorn
- Alcohol
- Sugars
- Vinegar (except apple cider vinegar)
- Coffee

The amount of food consumed can be an additional factor to consider. A 2013 study from Albert Einstein College of Medicine revealed that eating large amounts of food, or what is called caloric excess, can induce persistent inflammation, disrupt metabolic homeostasis, and contribute to a list of disorders that include obesity, diabetes, and insulin resistance. The Blue Zones study by National Geographic found that centurions who lived to be 100 years and older had a similar practice of pushing away from the table when they felt 80 percent full. The old adage about finishing everything on your plate is advice from another era that appears to be more detrimental than helpful in today's modern world.

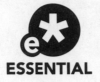

ESSENTIAL

Keeping a healthy attitude about following any diet helps keep stress levels at a minimum. Doing the best that you can and always working to do better bit by bit can be the most effective way to establish a solid foundation of health. Humans are creatures of habit and poor dietary habits can take a while to transform. Be kind to yourself along the way.

The length of time that individuals follow this diet can be determined by the health condition they're dealing with, or simply by a desire to maximize performance and vitality in their body. Almost every disease or condition has inflammation associated with it and can benefit from the autoimmune diet. In addition to using it with autoimmune diseases, it can also be used with cancers, candida, recent exposures to chemicals and heavy metals, or even a simple cold. Everyone can benefit by following it to one degree or another.

The more chronic or serious a condition is, the longer the length of the diet. Some people follow this diet permanently with great results.

CHAPTER 9

Functional Cooking

The art of cooking and food preparation takes on a new perspective when addressing autoimmune and other diseases. Everything that goes into creating a meal provides an opportunity to create greater health. Consideration of all the ingredients being used can increase one's awareness of the vital link between foods and health. The more aware you are of what you eat, the more conscious you are of your health. Fortunately, Mother Nature has blessed us with an immense variety of natural foods and plants to ensure that no meal has to be boring, and every meal can be healing.

Adopting a Gluten-Free Lifestyle

Adopting a gluten-free lifestyle shouldn't be looked upon as an unjust sentence that singles you out from friends, family, or coworkers. A more accurate point of view is that individuals who decide to add to their quality of life by going gluten-free are placing themselves in a unique position whereby they can enjoy their life with greater levels of health, vitality, endurance, vibrancy, happiness, and longevity.

In 2014, a team of Australian researchers found that a gluten-free diet improved mental function in celiac patients following a gluten-free diet. Italian researchers found that gluten-free diets also helped decrease intestinal damage. In 2011, another team of Italian researchers found that even in the absence of the gluten antibodies commonly found with gluten intolerance, markers for inflammation in the intestinal tract and in the blood both decreased.

According to the *New England Journal of Medicine*, gluten can cause over fifty-five diseases. Some of the major diseases on the list include cancer, schizophrenia, multiple sclerosis, anemia, depression, migraines, autism, and a long list of autoimmune diseases.

Gluten-free diet studies have also shown decreased body weight, improved blood sugar regulation, and decreased inflammation. Beyond celiac disease, gluten-free diets are also being used for skin conditions, neurological disorders, rheumatoid arthritis, diabetes, and HIV-associated disorders.

Gluten-free foods alone will not correct many autoimmune issues, and indeed many of the processed gluten-free foods often convert to sugars rapidly in the body. The elevation of blood sugar levels is problematic for autoimmune conditions. Gluten-free is not the answer to everything, but it's beginning to look like a key part of the puzzle. Learning the basics is the best way to get started and get healthy!

Getting Started

Eliminating foods that contain wheat, rye, and barley is the first step. For many people, that eliminates most forms of bread and pasta that they are used to eating. This creates the added benefit of reducing foods that quickly raise blood sugar, suppress immunity, and create inflammation.

Reading labels and becoming familiar with products that contain and don't contain gluten is next. There are several websites that post extensive lists on these products. A good place to start is the Gluten Intolerance Group at *www.gluten.org*. There, you can also find menus, restaurant lists, and even a list of drugs that contain gluten, something not often considered.

ALERT

Gluten sensitivities can range from mild and asymptomatic to severe and life threatening. Reactions to gluten may last a day or so in less sensitive individuals to weeks and months in people with celiac and gluten intolerance. If you're not sure about reactions to gluten, there are tests available such as those from Cyrex Laboratories and Enter-oLab that can help determine your status.

Throw out everything that contains gluten and gluten by-products. Start shopping for only those foods that are labeled gluten-free, as well as only those foods that work on an autoimmune diet. There's plenty to choose from. As you learn more and more about what foods will help create health and those that will detract from it, you'll be able to turn your kitchen into a healing sanctuary.

While creating wonderful meals at home is probably the best way to guarantee that you're getting the best of what you need, thousands of restaurants are now offering gluten-free foods on their menus, including over 150 fast-food chain restaurants all across America. Maintaining a gluten-free lifestyle is relatively easy today.

Hidden Gluten

It would be easy if avoiding foods with wheat, barley, and rye were all that was needed to ensure gluten-free success, but gluten is hidden in many foods that may not be so obvious. Learning what these hidden sources are is a part of the gluten-free lifestyle.

Some of the more common hidden sources include:

- Condiments
- Sauces (soy, barbecue)
- Chewing gums
- Salad dressings
- Malt vinegar
- Premade soups
- Premade marinades
- Meat substitutes
- Starch
- Instant coffee

The Celiac Disease Foundation website also lists other considerations that aren't normally thought of such as:

- Lipstick, lip gloss, and lip balms
- Herbal or nutritional supplements
- Drugs and over-the-counter medications
- Vitamins and mineral supplements
- Communion wafers

Additionally, the website mentions that there are cross-contamination issues that are more likely to be present in restaurants that prepare both gluten and gluten-free foods. When sticking to ordering primarily whole foods, many of these sources are eliminated.

QUESTION

Do foods that are labeled gluten-free contain zero amounts of gluten?
According to the final rule of the FDA in America, foods labeled gluten-free must contain less than 20 ppm (parts per million). Many gluten-free foods contain less than 5 or 10 ppm. Read labels for accurate information.

When following an autoimmune diet protocol, the majority of hidden gluten sources are not present. Be conscious of what you're eating. The closer a food is to its whole food form, the less likely it is that you'll run into problems.

Low-Histamine Foods

Eating foods that are high in histamine, when illness and inflammation are present, is like walking into a dynamite factory with a fiery torch. You could possibly make it in and out without creating a problem, but chances are that you won't. Once you do create a problem, it usually spreads and multiplies quite quickly and can have long-lasting effects. If eating foods creates allergic responses such as rashes, headaches, itching, cramping, or vomiting, the histamine levels in foods may be to blame.

Low-histamine foods, or foods without histamine, are a much better way to help keep the fires of inflammation at bay. While there is no universal food that would never create an allergic histamine response, as any one food could potentially be the source of allergic reactions in select individuals, there are foods low in histamine that make for wiser food selection choices.

The autoimmune diet is one that should consist primarily of fresh food products. Stick to fresh foods, as aging of foods tends to increase the levels of histamine in the foods. This can add to levels of inflammation in the body when these foods are consumed.

Fermented Foods

Fermented foods have a long history of benefits and can work very well under many conditions. Unfortunately, these foods tend to be high in histamine, which can make them a bad choice on an autoimmune diet. In many cases, it may be best to just leave them off entirely, but there may be another solution for some people who wish to take advantage of them.

FACT

The process of fermentation is ancient, extending back over 8,000 years. Fermented foods are considered to be the first probiotics due to the growth and use of bacteria during fermentation. Fermentation helps to predigest nutrients in foods, as well as playing a role in food safety and preservation. Fermented foods have great potential in health when they are well tolerated.

Anaerobic fermentation methods avoid creating the histamines that typical fermentation methods create. *Anaerobic* means "without oxygen." One company, Pickl-It (*www.Pickl-It.com*), has designed fermentation jars to create and maintain an anaerobic state of fermentation. This process helps eliminate the production of histamines in fermented foods. In combination with beneficial lactic acid bacteria, the Pickl-It jars help lock in vitamins, minerals, and nutrients that could otherwise be destroyed by other fermentation methods. For those who hate to give up fermented foods, try the Pickl-It jars and see if fermented foods will work for you on an autoimmune diet.

Canned Foods

Canned foods can have a tendency to ferment and therefore tend to be high in histamine. Whether it's fruit, veggies, fish, or meats, the decomposition and aging process of foods increases the levels of histamine. Stick to fresh foods for the best results.

Smoked Meats

Many people enjoy smoked meats, such as salmon, jerky, and pastrami, but they don't work well on an autoimmune diet. Like canned foods, the processing of the meats creates a maturation process that increases histamine. Choose fresh foods for greater health.

Histamine Promoters

In addition to foods that are high in histamine, some other foods may stimulate the release of histamine from immune cells in the body. There are some common foods that have been identified, but any food could cause this reaction based on your body's individual response to the food. Some of the foods to watch, but not necessarily avoid, include:

- Tomatoes
- Strawberries
- Pumpkin
- Papayas
- Pineapple
- Mangoes

- Raspberries
- Tangerines
- Grapefruit
- Shellfish
- Egg whites

If you think any of these foods is problematic for you, it may be that it is stimulating the release of histamine. As you heal the body, these types of reactions can lessen and disappear.

Resistant Starches

Resistant starches are foods that are known more for their ability to feed the bacteria of the colon, as digestion of them in the stomach and small intestine rarely occurs. Resistant starch foods tend to have a higher amount of fiber, but can include less seemingly fibrous varieties such as green bananas and raw potatoes.

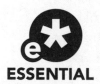

ESSENTIAL

Eating a wide variety of plant foods weekly can help increase fiber intake and greater diversity of the bacterial flora. Greater bacterial flora diversity is associated with greater levels of health. The fatty acids produced from fermentation of fibers has been associated with an increased production of white blood cells that help decrease inflammation.

Resistant starches act as prebiotics. Prebiotics are foods that feed the bacteria of the body, often referred to as probiotics when taken as a dietary supplement. When the bacteria of the body digest or ferment the resistant starches in foods, they create fatty acids that help reduce inflammation and protect the lining of the entire intestinal tract. These acids include acetate, propionate, and butyrate acids. This can help prevent the condition known as leaky gut, whereby food particles enter the circulation and create inflammation and allergic responses.

A lack of enough fermentable fibers, like those found in resistant starches, has been associated with an increased risk of diseases of the colon by researchers from the United Kingdom and Australia. Without enough carbohydrates, the composition of the bacterial flora changes toward a profile that is more prone to inflammation. Resistant starch isn't feeding you so much as it's feeding the garden within you.

ALERT

Some people have trouble with higher amounts of resistant starch in their diet due to its ability to temporarily increase the production of gas. This effect usually goes away within a week or so, as the ratios of bacteria in the gut change. Starting out with smaller amounts is helpful. Correcting imbalances in the gut with a candida diet first can help avoid problems.

One can increase and create resistant starches in some foods by cooking them first and then refrigerating them overnight before eating them. Foods that fall into this category include potatoes, brown rice, and pasta. By following this method of preparation, one can increase the amount of resistant starch and decrease the effect on blood sugars. One study showed that using this method with pasta and then reheating the pasta further decreased the sugar content. Potatoes, rice, and pasta aren't typically included as food choices on many autoimmune diet lists. Converting them to resistant starches can change their effect on the body and make them a part of an autoimmune diet.

The Secrets of Spices

The common spice rack can be as important to health as the common medicine cabinet, and typically a lot safer. Spices have played an important part in the history of the world, as countries have attempted to control their trade and fought wars over them. Spices have long been sought out for their magical, mystical powers, especially for their healing properties. The use of spices and herbs as healing agents has been practiced for thousands of years and continues to this day.

Many spices have anti-inflammatory properties that make them an excellent choice for autoimmune diets. These include cinnamon, cloves, ginger, turmeric, garlic, cayenne, black pepper, and others. Peppers are a part of the nightshade family and may not work for some people but work well for others. Their ability to reduce inflammation can offset any inflammatory effect that they might possess.

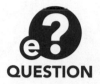

QUESTION

Is there one spice or herb that can help me more than the rest?
Consulting with a doctor is the best way to determine what might work for anyone best, but if there were one herb or spice that has been proven to benefit more conditions than any other, it would be turmeric. There are over 7,300 peer-reviewed studies on turmeric's benefits.

The best way to buy and store spices is to buy spices whole and grind them when you're ready to use them. Many stores have spices that have been sitting around for months or years. Check with ethnic markets or spice merchants, where spices tend to be fresher and sold at a much faster rate due to their popularity. Store them in glass jars when you get them home to keep them fresher longer and to seal out other odors.

You can also check your local famers' markets for fresh herbs, instead of dried ones, or grow your own. Use them fresh, or dry them out and then use them. Remember, fresher is better. Buying spices in smaller quantities will help ensure that they don't get stale. As you discover which spices work best for your condition and which ones you like to cook and flavor foods with, you'll know which ones to buy more of.

Don't be afraid to experiment with spices. The average American only uses one or two spices on a daily basis, while the average Indian uses eleven. Using spices in combination can increase the benefits, but avoid buying premixes, as they can contain gluten and higher levels of histamine. Spice up your life and your health!

Meal Planning for Long-Term Health

Now that you have the basics and understand much more about autoimmune conditions and diets, it's a good time to take a look at meal planning.

You'll want to create a grocery list that you can refer to when shopping. For those people into using their smartphones, there are several apps available that will provide shopping lists, as well as restaurant recommendations, brand names, and guide maps to help you navigate more than just the local grocery store aisle.

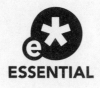

ESSENTIAL

One way to ensure success is by taking the time to sit down and plan out your meals for the week. This helps you create a shopping list of what you'll need. Then you can determine where you'll need to shop to pick up the necessary supplies. Farmers' markets are a good place to pick up fresh organic whole foods.

Keeping meals as fresh as possible means that you could be shopping a bit more than you may be used to. It also means that the nutrient level of the foods you're eating is bound to increase, as there's no comparison between fresh foods and processed foods. In fact, processed foods are so devoid of nutrients, they always have to have the nutrients added.

Planning for Success

Meal planning means that you'll need to assess your strengths and weaknesses when it comes to preparing yourself meals throughout the week. Strengthening your weak areas and maximizing your strengths will help ensure success. If your schedule on some days doesn't allow for a lot of food preparation, plan accordingly or make reservations at a gluten-free restaurant for that time. Go with what works for you.

If eating out frequently doesn't work well for the budget, stick to simple meals with a variety of spices and herbs that enhance the flavors. Pick up some cookbooks with simple recipes that you can modify easily, if needed. There are several dozen gluten-free cookbooks available, as well as a variety of websites and videos on cooking. With meal planning, you'll be focusing primarily on meats, vegetables, and some fruit.

ALERT

If you're diabetic, hypoglycemic, or have insulin resistance, keeping your blood sugar balanced is very important in overcoming autoimmune diseases. Blood sugar imbalances create high levels of inflammation, and diabetes is often associated with other autoimmune diseases. Correcting your diet and maintaining constant levels of blood sugar are very important. Consult your doctor about using supplements, herbs, or medications that can help you.

If you're experiencing blood sugar imbalances, you'll need to restrict the fruit a little more and eat primarily low-glycemic fruit. Dr. Datis Kharrazian, DC, who specializes in autoimmune thyroid disorders and a number of other conditions linked to autoimmunity, recommends low-glycemic fruit such as apples, apricots, avocados, berries, cherries, grapefruit, lemons, oranges, peaches, pears, plums. Eating fruit that isn't quite ripe yet is a good rule to follow. Sour or slightly sour is a good taste range to aim for.

Ask for Help

Many people try to go it alone when they don't need to. Ask friends, family, and others for ideas on cooking and preparing meals. Let people know that you're trying out a new way of eating to maximize your health and achieve your body's true potential. Most people are pleasantly surprised to find out how many people are already eating along these lines. Soon, you'll have an abundance of ideas and probably a few free meals along the way. The nature of humans is to help one another, especially when it comes to eating. Eating together with others is a great way to socialize and find out more ideas.

A New Beginning

The lists of foods presented here won't work for everyone. The autoimmune diet goes beyond just eating gluten-free and incorporates several other dietary recommendations that are aimed at addressing inflammation. Gluten-free eating alone can have many benefits, but it might not be able to afford complete relief of symptoms.

For some people, addressing systemic fungal candida first will help bring back order and balance to the intestinal tract, where many autoimmune conditions are believed to originate. This can serve as an excellent foundation from which to build upon by then following it up with the auto-immune diet.

ESSENTIAL

A good candida diet will follow along the lines of an autoimmune diet. It will help balance and improve the immune system, detoxify the body, correct fungal candida back to its normal yeast form, and help restore normal, healthy body flora. Additionally, it will help improve the health of the gut, balance blood sugar responses, and decrease inflammation.

Consider this book to be a starting point, a launch pad from which you can develop and refine what works for you. There's no need to create a hard-line dogma, as the variations in diet will allow you to make your diet a living testament of what works and doesn't work for your body. Play around with recipes, foods, supplements, and everything else presented here. If something mentioned here doesn't work for you, don't eat it. Each failure defines what doesn't work and helps keep you on track with what does work. In that sense, everything creates a win.

No one knows you better than you do. No one can help you more than you can help yourself. No one else can be who you are. This book provides an outline that anyone can follow. Use it as a tool to become the best that you can be. Best wishes on your success!

CHAPTER 10

Breakfast

Bite-Sized Smoked Salmon
Frittatas
152

Fluffy Yellow Turmeric
Scrambled Eggs
153

Spicy Zucchini Egg Scramble
154

Turkey Breakfast Sausages
155

Farmer's Egg Casserole
156

Salvadoran *Huevos Picados con
Ejotes* (Green Bean Scramble)
157

The Perfect Breakfast Potatoes
158

Crustless Spinach and Potato
Quiche
159

Spicy Kale Scramble
160

Breakfast Fried Rice
161

Resistant Starch Porridge
162

Sweet Start Breakfast Porridge
162

Poached Eggs and Porridge
163

Protein Power Breakfast
164

Brown Rice Frittata
164

Bite-Sized Smoked Salmon Frittatas

A fun and healthy way of making frittatas, these are easy to store in the fridge and always delicious.

INGREDIENTS | MAKES 20 MINI FRITTATAS

4 large eggs

¼ cup light coconut milk

Salt to taste

¼ teaspoon freshly ground black pepper

3 ounces shredded smoked salmon

¼ cup chopped fresh dill

Variation

You can replace the dill with chopped fresh parsley or replace salmon with turkey bacon.

1. Preheat the oven to 375°F. Spray a 24-cup mini muffin tin with nonstick spray.

2. In a medium bowl, whisk together the eggs, coconut milk, salt, and pepper.

3. Add the salmon and dill. Mix well.

4. Fill the prepared muffin tin cups ¾ full with the mixture.

5. Bake for 7–10 minutes or until a toothpick inserted into the center of a frittata comes out clean.

6. Remove from the oven and loosen the frittatas with a rubber spatula. Enjoy warm or cold.

Fluffy Yellow Turmeric Scrambled Eggs

This is a milk-free, but no less delicious, version of the classic dish.

INGREDIENTS | SERVES 2

2 tablespoons extra virgin olive oil

4 large eggs

¼ cup light coconut milk

½ teaspoon ground turmeric

Salt and freshly ground black pepper to taste

Yellow Color

The yellow color will be added by the turmeric, which is also an excellent anti-inflammatory spice.

1. In a large skillet over medium heat, heat up the oil.

2. In a medium bowl, whisk together the eggs, coconut milk, turmeric, salt, and pepper.

3. Add the eggs to the hot oil and slowly scramble using a rubber spatula. Stir every 20 seconds.

4. Cook for about 3 minutes or until the eggs reach the desired texture.

Spicy Zucchini Egg Scramble

This is a favorite breakfast dish for those who desire a spicy kick in the morning. The cayenne pepper is used as a natural painkiller and anti-inflammatory.

INGREDIENTS | SERVES 2

2 tablespoons olive oil

1 medium zucchini, diced

Salt and freshly ground black pepper to taste

Pinch cayenne pepper, or to taste

4 large eggs

1. In a large skillet over medium heat, heat up the olive oil.

2. Add the zucchini and sauté until brown and soft, about 3 minutes.

3. Season the zucchini with salt, pepper, and cayenne pepper.

4. Add the eggs one at a time.

5. Scramble the eggs using a rubber spatula. If desired, add more salt to taste.

6. Cook for about 3–5 minutes, until the eggs are cooked to the desired doneness. Enjoy warm.

Turkey Breakfast Sausages

Since turkey is a leaner protein, you can use chicken if you prefer a juicer sausage. Enjoy these sausages with scrambled eggs for a delicious and filling breakfast.

INGREDIENTS | MAKES 10–12 PATTIES

2 pounds ground turkey

2 teaspoons salt

1 teaspoon freshly ground black pepper

2 teaspoons ground cumin

1 teaspoon cayenne pepper

4 teaspoons chili powder

2 teaspoons Herbes de Provence

1 clove garlic, minced

2 tablespoons olive oil

1 large egg

1. Preheat the oven to 350°F.

2. In a large bowl, combine all the ingredients and mix well with your hands; you can wear gloves if desired.

3. After all the ingredients are well combined, form into thin 4"-diameter patties.

4. Place the patties in a large baking dish. Bake for 20–25 minutes, until browned.

Make It a Burger

You may use this recipe to make a turkey burger. Simply make the patties into bigger burger-sized patties.

Farmer's Egg Casserole

This is the perfect way to start your day if you're looking for a protein-rich meal.

INGREDIENTS | SERVES 6–8

1 tablespoon olive oil

1 pound lean ground beef (10–15% fat)

2 teaspoons salt, divided

1 teaspoon freshly ground black pepper, divided

½ cup chopped onion

½ cup diced fresh green beans

¼ cup chopped mushrooms

12 large eggs

1 cup light coconut milk

¼ teaspoon dried rosemary

Milk Alternatives

You may replace the coconut milk with almond milk if you prefer. If you can't find light coconut milk, use ½ cup full-fat coconut milk and ½ cup of water and mix them together.

1. Preheat the oven to 350°F. Grease a 9" × 13" baking pan.

2. In a large skillet over medium heat, heat the olive oil.

3. Add the ground beef to the skillet and season with 1 teaspoon salt and ½ teaspoon black pepper. Cook the ground beef until browned and halfway cooked, about 5 minutes.

4. Add the onions, green beans, and mushrooms. Cook for 7 minutes, stirring occasionally until the green beans are al dente.

5. Remove from the heat and let cool for 10 minutes.

6. In a large bowl, combine the eggs, coconut milk, rosemary, and remaining salt and pepper. Whisk together until the eggs are fully blended.

7. Add the beef and vegetable mixture to the eggs and whisk together.

8. Pour the mixture into the prepared baking pan and bake for 30–35 minutes.

Salvadoran *Huevos Picados con Ejotes* (Green Bean Scramble)

This is a simple and delicious recipe, commonly eaten in the small Central American country of El Salvador.

INGREDIENTS | SERVES 4

2 tablespoons olive oil

1 cup fresh green beans cut into ¼"
pieces

¼ cup chopped white onion

Salt and freshly ground black pepper to
taste

8 large eggs

Sliced green onions, for garnish

Make It Fun and Colorful!

Make this dish fun and appealing to kids by
combining purple, white, and green beans.

1. In a large skillet over medium heat, heat up the olive oil.

2. Add the green beans and onions and sauté for 5 minutes or until soft. Season with salt and pepper.

3. Add the eggs one at a time, and season the eggs with salt and pepper. Using a rubber spatula, scramble the eggs. Cook the eggs for about 4 minutes or until they have reached the desire doneness.

4. Serve the eggs garnished with green onions.

The Perfect Breakfast Potatoes

These flavorful potatoes will work perfect with your favorite omelet or scramble.

INGREDIENTS | SERVES 4

4 cups water

1 teaspoon salt, plus extra to taste

6 medium yellow potatoes cut into 1"
  cubes

3 tablespoons olive oil

1½ tablespoons Herbes de Provence

Freshly ground black pepper to taste

Yellow Potatoes

Yellow potatoes are a popular choice for their soft and creamy texture, but you can use your favorite potatoes if you don't have yellow potatoes available. Russet potatoes are starchier but will also work great with this recipe.

1. In a large stockpot, bring the water to a boil and add 1 teaspoon salt.

2. Add the potatoes, cover, and cook over medium to low heat for approximately 7 minutes. (You are trying to precook the potatoes; you don't want them too soft, just enough to be al dente.)

3. Strain the potatoes.

4. In a large skillet over medium heat, heat the oil.

5. Add the potatoes and immediately season with Herbes de Provence, salt, and pepper to taste. Stir and make sure every potato is covered with seasonings.

6. Cook the potatoes until they have a brown crust on every corner, stirring every minute or so. This process takes about 10 minutes.

7. Refrigerate the potatoes overnight to make them a resistance starch.

Crustless Spinach and Potato Quiche

This is a perfect recipe to make ahead of time and then refrigerate or freeze until you need it.

INGREDIENTS | SERVES 4–6

1 tablespoon olive oil

1 large shallot, chopped

1 (10-ounce) package frozen chopped spinach, thawed and drained

6 large eggs, beaten

½ teaspoon salt, or more to taste

½ teaspoon freshly ground black pepper

1 cup cubed Resistant Starch Potatoes (see recipe in Chapter 11)

Rice Variation

To give it a different texture, try replacing the potatoes with Resistant Starch Brown Rice (see recipe in Chapter 11). You may also use half potatoes and half rice.

1. Preheat the oven to 350°F. Lightly grease a 9" pan.

2. In a large skillet over medium heat, heat the oil. Add the shallots and cook until translucent approximately 4 minutes.

3. Stir in the spinach and continue cooking until most of the water has been evaporated. Remove from heat and let cool for 4 minutes.

4. In a medium bowl, combine the eggs, salt, and pepper and potatoes.

5. Add the spinach to the eggs and potato mixture and stir to blend. Pour the egg and spinach mixture into the prepared baking pan.

6. Bake until the eggs have set, about 25–30 minutes. Let cool for approximately 8 minutes before serving. This will help the eggs solidify.

Spicy Kale Scramble

This is a great post-workout breakfast, providing healthy proteins and a healthy amount of greens.

INGREDIENTS | SERVES 1

1 tablespoon olive oil

1 cup chopped kale

3 large eggs

2 teaspoons turmeric

Salt and freshly ground black pepper to taste

Pinch cayenne pepper

Add More Greens

Feel free to add your favorite greens to this recipe. Spinach, arugula, and collard greens work great!

1. In a medium skillet over medium heat, heat the oil.

2. Add the kale and cook, stirring constantly, for 3 minutes. Add the eggs one at a time, or beat the eggs prior to adding them, this will give a fluffier texture.

3. Immediately add the turmeric, salt, pepper, and cayenne pepper.

4. Scramble the eggs and kale.

5. Cook until the eggs are fully cooked; this process takes 3–4 minutes. Serve immediately.

Breakfast Fried Rice

This breakfast version of the Asian classic makes the perfect dish when you need a healthy serving of carbs and protein. This dish also works great with cubed zucchini, green beans, or other vegetables of your choice.

INGREDIENTS | SERVES 2

1 tablespoon olive oil

6 large eggs

Salt and freshly ground black pepper to taste

1 cup Resistant Starch Brown Rice (see recipe in Chapter 11)

Pinch cayenne pepper

2 teaspoons lemon juice

1. In a medium skillet over medium heat, heat the oil.

2. Add the eggs one at a time and season with salt and pepper.

3. Scramble the eggs and cook for 1–2 minutes; the eggs will still be raw.

4. Add the rice and scramble together with the eggs. Add more salt and pepper to the rice and egg mixture. Cook for 2–3 minutes, until the rice is hot.

5. Sprinkle with cayenne pepper, and stir the mixture.

6. Squeeze some lemon juice on the top and serve warm.

Resistant Starch Porridge

The steps in this recipe can be followed for any porridge recipe.

INGREDIENTS | SERVES 4

3 cups water

¼ teaspoon salt

1 cup brown rice cereal or brown rice farina

Hot Brown Rice Cereal

Whenever this book refers to brown rice cereal, it is referring to the type of cereal that needs to be cooked before eating. In this recipe the rice must be refrigerated overnight before eating; this process changes the starch in the rice to a resistant starch.

1. In a medium pot bring the water to a boil.

2. Add the salt and the cereal.

3. Reduce the heat to low and cook the rice cereal for 6–8 minutes, stirring occasionally.

4. Turn off heat, and let cool for 15 minutes.

5. Transfer the cereal to the refrigerator and refrigerate overnight.

6. The next day, your cereal is ready to be reheated with a little water.

Sweet Start Breakfast Porridge

Here is a sweet breakfast porridge that is a favorite among fruit lovers or anyone who wants a delicious start to their day.

INGREDIENTS | SERVES 1

½ cup Resistant Starch Porridge (see recipe in this chapter)

2 tablespoons water

¼ medium banana, sliced

¼ cup blueberries

¼ cup diced apple

1 teaspoon ground cinnamon

Kick It Up with Coconut Milk

If you don't have any reactions to pure coconut milk, which should only contain coconut cream and water, then feel free to add some to this recipe.

1. In a small pot over medium-low heat, warm up the porridge and water. Stir, and add more water if needed. The porridge should be soft and warm, not too lumpy.

2. In a small bowl, combine the fruit and cinnamon. Mix all the fruit together until all pieces are coated with cinnamon.

3. Pour the hot porridge into a serving bowl. Add the fruit mixture on top.

4. Stir the fruit with the porridge and enjoy.

Poached Eggs and Porridge

Not everyone likes sweet in the morning, so here is a savory way to enjoy brown rice porridge with a creamy poached egg.

INGREDIENTS | SERVES 1

1 cup plus 2 tablespoons water

¼ cup Resistant Starch Porridge (see recipe in this chapter)

¼ teaspoon salt, plus extra to taste

2 teaspoons coconut oil

2 large eggs

¼ teaspoon smoked paprika

1. In a medium saucepan bring 1 cup of water to a boil.

2. In a separate small pot over low heat, warm up the porridge with the 2 tablespoons water, ¼ teaspoon salt, and coconut oil.

3. Meanwhile, crack 1 egg into a small bowl.

4. Slowly and gently slip the egg into the boiling water. Repeat the process for the second egg.

5. Cover the pan, and let the water boil over low heat for 1 minute.

6. Turn off heat and let the eggs cook for another 3 minutes with the heat off and the pan covered.

7. Using a slotted spoon, immediately remove the eggs one at a time and serve over the hot porridge.

8. Sprinkle smoked paprika and a little salt on top.

Protein Power Breakfast

This recipe contains over 22 grams of protein and is the perfect breakfast for any athlete or an excellent meal at any time of the day.

INGREDIENTS | SERVES 1

1 tablespoon olive oil
¼ pound (10% fat) ground beef
Salt and freshly ground black pepper to taste
½ medium zucchini, chopped
¼ cup Resistant Starch Brown Rice (see recipe in Chapter 11)
2 large eggs
½ medium avocado, sliced

1. In a medium skillet over medium heat, heat the olive oil.

2. Add the ground beef and season it with salt and pepper. Cook about 4 minutes, stirring occasionally.

3. Add the zucchini and cook for 2 minutes or until soft.

4. Add the brown rice and stir for about 3 minutes, until the rice is hot.

5. Add the eggs one at a time, season with salt and pepper, and scramble. Cook until the eggs have reached the desired doneness.

6. Serve the scramble in a bowl. Garnish with the sliced avocado on top.

Brown Rice Frittata

A frittata is the Italian version of the American omelet. The brown rice gives it a nice chewy texture.

INGREDIENTS | SERVES 1

3 large eggs
¼ cup Resistant Starch Brown Rice (see recipe in Chapter 11)
1 tablespoon chopped fresh basil
Salt and freshly ground black pepper to taste
1 tablespoon olive oil

1. In a medium bowl, mix the eggs, rice, basil, salt, and pepper. Whisk together all the ingredients.

2. In an 8" pan over medium heat, heat the oil.

3. Add the egg mixture to the pan and cover. Cook for about 3 minutes, until the eggs are almost set.

4. Flip the frittata and cook for another 3 minutes.

5. Serve immediately. Garnish with extra chopped basil if desired.

Try It with Different Herbs!

Try this recipe with your favorite herbs. Italian parsley works great or regular parsley works just great if Italian isn't available.

CHAPTER 11

Lunch

Resistant Starch Brown Rice
166

Resistant Starch Brown
Rice Pasta
167

Resistant Starch Potatoes
168

Mediterranean Turkey Burger
168

Tortilla Española (Spanish
Omelet)
169

Herbes de Provence–Crusted
Bison Sirloin Tip
170

Sunny California Beet Salad
171

Harvest Chicken Soup
172

Beet and Peach Salad
173

Egglicious Beet Salad
174

Ojai Ginger Lemon Salmon
175

Peruvian Ceviche
176

Pollo Verde (Green Chicken)
177

Cauliflower and Potatoes
(*Aloo Gobi*)
177

Chicken and Cauliflower Stir-Fry
178

Chicken Breasts with Capers
179

Halibut with Olives and Arugula
179

Olive and Capers Pasta
180

Resistant Starch Brown Rice

This simple rice recipe will be the base for other recipes to follow. Brown rice must be refrigerated overnight to counteract the inflammatory effects found in grains.

INGREDIENTS | SERVES 8–10

1 tablespoon olive oil

1 tablespoon coconut oil

2 cups short-grain brown rice soaked in water overnight and drained

4 cups water

1 teaspoon salt

The Cooling Process

The process of cooking the brown rice and letting it cool overnight changes the starches in the rice to a resistant starch. Resistant starches are excellent for their anti-inflammatory properties.

1. In a medium saucepan over medium heat, heat the oils.

2. Add the drained rice and cook for 5 minutes, stirring frequently until the rice begins to crack and changes to a light brown color.

3. Add the water and salt. Reduce the heat to low, cover the rice, and cook for 40–45 minutes, or until the water has been completely absorbed.

4. Turn off the heat and let it cool.

5. Place the rice in the fridge overnight. The rice will be ready to be eaten plain or used in recipes.

Resistant Starch Brown Rice Pasta

This pasta recipe is used with other recipes found in this book.

INGREDIENTS | SERVES 2

4½ quarts water

1 teaspoon salt

1 tablespoon olive oil

1 (12-ounce) package brown rice pasta

The Cooling Process

The process of cooking the brown rice pasta and then letting it cool overnight changes the starches in the pasta to a resistant starch. Resistant starches do not promote inflammation in the body. Eating the brown rice pasta right after cooking it may promote inflammation.

1. Bring the water to a boil in a large pot over medium heat.

2. Add the salt, oil, and pasta.

3. Cook, stirring occasionally, for 15 minutes or until the pasta is cooked to the desired doneness.

4. Remove the pasta from heat, and let it cool down.

5. Transfer the pasta to the refrigerator and leave overnight. The pasta is now ready to be used in different dishes.

Resistant Starch Potatoes

These potatoes make a delicious potato salad. Use your favorite homemade mayonnaise and herbs to make a delicious and healthy lunch or side dish!

INGREDIENTS | SERVES 4

4½ quarts water

1 teaspoon salt

1 tablespoon olive oil

3 large potatoes of your choice peeled and cut into 1" cubes

1. Bring the water to a boil in a large pot over medium heat.

2. Add the salt, oil, and potatoes. Cook for 20–25 minutes or until the potatoes are cooked to the desired doneness.

3. Remove the potatoes from the heat and let cool down for about 20 minutes.

4. Transfer the potatoes to the refrigerator and leave overnight. The potatoes are now ready to be used in different dishes.

Mediterranean Turkey Burger

This is a delicious recipe for those who don't like to eat beef. Try this burger over a Greek salad.

INGREDIENTS | SERVES 4

1 pound ground turkey

3 tablespoons extra virgin olive oil, divided

1 tablespoon turmeric

2 teaspoons ground cumin

¼ cup finely chopped purple onion

1 clove garlic, crushed

1 cup chopped kalamata olives

¼ cup diced sun-dried tomatoes

1. In a medium bowl, mix the turkey, 2 tablespoons extra virgin olive oil, spices, and vegetables.

2. Form into 4 (¼-pound) patties. Brush the burgers with the remaining extra virgin olive oil.

3. Grill the burgers over medium heat for about 5 minutes per side, or until the internal temperature has reached at least 160°F.

4. Serve over salad and mashed potatoes if desired.

Tortilla Española (Spanish Omelet)

Not to be confused with the Mexican corn or wheat tortilla, this is a delicious and moist omelet that can be enjoyed at any time of the day.

INGREDIENTS | SERVES 2

2 tablespoons extra-virgin olive oil, divided

2 medium yellow potatoes, peeled and diced

½ medium yellow onion, diced

1½ teaspoons ground turmeric, divided

1 teaspoon sea salt, plus more to season potatoes

6 large eggs

1 teaspoon freshly ground black pepper

Variation

If you don't have reactions to nightshades you may add some bell peppers and diced tomatoes to this recipe.

1. In a 10" frying pan over medium heat, heat 1 tablespoon olive oil.

2. Add the diced potatoes and cook for 5 minutes, stirring occasionally.

3. Add the diced onion and season with ½ teaspoon turmeric and salt to taste. Cook until the onion is translucent and the potatoes are soft and fully cooked. This process takes approximately 5 minutes.

4. Remove the potato and onion mixture from the heat and let cool for 5 minutes.

5. Meanwhile, in a medium bowl whisk together the eggs, 1 teaspoon salt, pepper, and remaining turmeric. Whisk for 2 minutes.

6. Whisk in the cooled potato and onion mixture.

7. Using a separate 10" pan over medium heat, warm up the remaining tablespoon of olive oil and add the egg mixture.

8. Cover and cook for about 4 minutes on each side or until the eggs are fully cooked.

Herbes de Provence–Crusted Bison Sirloin Tip

Bison is a lean and healthy protein. Its nutritional content is similar to that of turkey.

INGREDIENTS | SERVES 2–3

2 teaspoons sea salt
1 teaspoon freshly ground black pepper
1 tablespoon Herbes de Provence
1 pound bison sirloin tip
1 tablespoon olive oil

Bison versus Turkey

A quarter pound of ground bison contains 10 grams of fat, 4 grams of saturated fat, and 29 grams of protein. Ground turkey contains 10.5 grams of fat, 3 grams of saturated fat, and just a little over 20 grams of protein.

1. Preheat the oven to 225°F.

2. In a small bowl, mix together the salt, pepper, and Herbes de Provence.

3. Meanwhile, place the bison in a medium baking pan.

4. Coat the bison with olive oil. (This will help the seasonings stick to the bison and help the browning process.)

5. Evenly rub the seasoning mixture all over the bison.

6. Heat up a large cast-iron skillet or grill pan over medium-high heat.

7. Place the bison in the hot skillet for 3–4 minutes per side. Return the bison to the baking pan.

8. Bake for 1 hour 35 minutes for medium rare, or until a thermometer reads 125°F interior temperature.

9. Turn off the oven and leave the roast in the oven for another 20 minutes.

10. Slice thinly and serve.

Sunny California Beet Salad

Beets are not only beautiful to the eye, but they are loaded with nutrients, antioxidants, and anti-inflammatory properties.

INGREDIENTS | SERVES 2

⅓ cup olive oil

¼ cup orange juice

2 tablespoons lemon juice

1 teaspoon salt, or more to taste

1 teaspoon freshly ground black pepper

1 tablespoon raw honey

Pinch cayenne pepper

3 medium red beets peeled, julienned or shredded

1 large carrot peeled, julienned or shredded

1½ cups julienned baby spinach

½ head napa cabbage, julienned

Be Creative with Your Options

This salad works great with most raw and chewy vegetables. If you desire more texture, try adding fresh pears, apples, purple cabbage, etc. The options are endless.

1. Make the vinaigrette: Place the oil, citrus juices, salt, pepper, honey, and cayenne pepper in a small bowl and whisk all together. You may blend them in a blender if you prefer.

2. Meanwhile, in a large bowl mix together all the julienned vegetables.

3. Pour the vinaigrette on the vegetables and toss using your hands or tongs.

4. Let the vegetables marinate for 3 minutes. Serve immediately.

Harvest Chicken Soup

This is a simple and delicious chicken soup. It provides the perfect amount of protein, vegetables, and starches to make a satisfying meal.

INGREDIENTS | SERVES 4

6 cups water

1 cup sliced carrots, skin on

1 cup sliced celery

3 bay leaves

1 clove garlic, mashed

Salt and freshly ground black pepper to taste

1½ pounds boneless, skinless chicken breasts, cut into cubes

1½ cups cubed yellow potatoes

1 cup green beans, cut into ½" slices

1 cup cubed zucchini

1 tablespoon ground turmeric

More Flavor!

For more flavor replace a portion of the chicken breast with a cut that contains more fat and bones. You may also replace half the water with a good-quality chicken stock.

1. In a large pot, bring the water to a boil.

2. Add the carrots, celery, bay leaves, garlic, salt, and pepper to the boiling water. Let simmer over medium heat for 10 minutes.

3. Add the chicken and let simmer over medium heat for 25 minutes covered.

4. Add the potatoes and green beans and re-cover with lid. Let cook for 10 minutes.

5. Once the potatoes are tender, add the zucchini and turmeric. (Zucchini cooks very quickly, so you always add this last.)

6. Check the soup for salt and add more if desired.

Beet and Peach Salad

Enjoy this fresh and juicy salad on a hot summer day.

INGREDIENTS | SERVES 2

6 medium red beets, tops and ends removed

2 large ripe peaches

10 fresh mint leaves

2 tablespoons olive oil

1 tablespoon lemon juice

Salt and freshly ground black pepper to taste

Boiling versus Roasting

If you are looking to get the most flavor and sweetness out of your beets, roasting is the best option. Roasting concentrates the flavors and sugars, while boiling cooks the beets faster.

1. Preheat the oven to 400°F. Wrap the individual beets in aluminum foil.

2. Roast for 25–30 minutes until a knife slips easily into the center of each beet.

3. Remove the beets from the oven, open the foil pouches, and let cool.

4. Meanwhile, cut the peaches into wedges.

5. Once cool, peel the beets and cut into quarters.

6. In a large bowl, combine the beets and peaches.

7. Chop the mint leaves and add to the bowl.

8. In a small bowl whisk together the oil, lemon juice, salt, and pepper.

9. Pour the dressing on the salad and toss, making sure that every piece is coated.

Egglicious Beet Salad

This delicious salad makes a decadent side dish for any holiday party.

INGREDIENTS | SERVES 4

6–8 large red beets, tops and ends removed

5 large eggs

3 tablespoons olive oil

1 tablespoon lemon juice

¼ teaspoon dry mustard

Salt and freshly ground black pepper to taste

1 tablespoon chopped chives

Play Around with Presentation

The shape of the eggs and beets make them excellent ingredients to play around with in the presentation. Try cutting them into round slices, then place a slice of beet at the bottom, follow by a slice of egg, and garnish with chives. Drizzle with a little bit of the dressing and serve them as hors d'oeuvres.

1. Preheat the oven to 400°F. Wrap the individual beets in aluminum foil.

2. Roast for 25–30 minutes, until a knife slips easily into the center of each beet.

3. Remove the beets from the oven, open the foil pouches, and let cool.

4. Bring 4 cups water to a boil and add the eggs. Boil the eggs for 10–12 minutes. Remove the eggs and transfer them immediately to ice water.

5. Peel the beets and cut into quarters.

6. Peel the eggs and cut into quarters.

7. In a small bowl, whisk together the oil, lemon juice, mustard, salt, and pepper.

8. Combine all the ingredients in a large bowl and mix. Enjoy immediately or refrigerate for up to 3 days.

Ojai Ginger Lemon Salmon

Enjoy this wonderful fish on top of mixed greens or steamed vegetables.

INGREDIENTS | SERVES 2

Zest of 1 large lemon

2 tablespoons lemon juice

3 tablespoons extra virgin olive oil, divided

2 tablespoons freshly grated gingerroot

½ teaspoon salt

½ teaspoon freshly ground black pepper

Pinch cayenne pepper

2 (8-ounce) salmon fillets

Bake It

You can also bake this dish. Simply bake the fillets after marinating them. Pan-frying, however, does give them a crispy texture.

1. In a medium bowl add lemon zest.

2. To the same bowl, add the lemon juice, 2 tablespoons olive oil, ginger, salt, pepper, and cayenne pepper. Mix well.

3. In a plastic bag or airtight container, add the salmon fillets and pour in the marinade.

4. Put in the refrigerator and let marinate for 3–4 hours, or if you prefer, overnight.

5. In a large frying pan over medium heat, heat up 1 tablespoon olive oil.

6. Place the salmon fillets flesh-side down in the pan and cook for 4–5 minutes.

7. Flip to the skin side and cook for 3–4 minutes until the skin is crispy.

8. Serve on a bed of your favorite salad.

Peruvian Ceviche

This is a modified version of the Peruvian classic. In the original Peruvian recipe a yellow pepper (aji amarillo) is used, but this recipe replaces it with jalapeño peppers.

INGREDIENTS | SERVES 2

2 (1-pound) whitefish fillets, preferably wild sea bass

2 teaspoons garlic paste

2 teaspoons salt, plus more to taste

1 teaspoon freshly ground black pepper

Juice of 5 large lemons

3 tablespoons finely chopped fresh cilantro

½ medium purple onion, sliced and soaked in water for 10 minutes

4 large iceberg lettuce wedges

1 medium sweet potato, peeled, boiled, and cooled

1. Cut the fish into small ½" cubes.

2. In a medium glass bowl, add the fish and garlic paste.

3. Add the salt and stir to make sure all pieces are covered. Add the pepper and stir.

4. Add the lemon juice, stir, and let the fish marinate (cook) for 5 minutes.

5. Add the cilantro and onion and let marinate in the juice for 5 more minutes. The ceviche is now ready to be served.

6. Serve on a bed of lettuce leaves and chunks of boiled sweet potatoes.

Raw Fish Warning

Because this recipe contains raw fish you should use only fresh fish from a reputable source.

Pollo Verde (Green Chicken)

The base of this recipe is cilantro. This magnificent herb is well known for its ability to assist the body in eliminating heavy metals. Enjoy this recipe on top of Resistant Starch Brown Rice (see recipe in this chapter).

INGREDIENTS | SERVES 4

1 cup gluten-free chicken stock

2 bunches fresh cilantro, about 3 cups chopped

Juice of 2 large lemons

½ medium white onion

1 clove garlic

3 tablespoons olive oil

1 tablespoon salt, or more to taste

2 teaspoons freshly ground black pepper

1½ pounds boneless, skinless chicken breast tenders

1. Preheat the oven to 350°F.

2. In a blender combine the chicken stock, cilantro, lemon juice, onion, garlic, oil, salt, and pepper. Add more salt if needed.

3. Place the chicken tenders in a large baking pan. Pour the marinade on top of the chicken, cover with plastic wrap, and let marinate for 30 minutes in the fridge.

4. Bake for 40–45 minutes.

Cauliflower and Potatoes (*Aloo Gobi*)

This Indian recipe can be enjoyed as a meal or as a side dish.

INGREDIENTS | SERVES 4

1 tablespoon garlic paste

1 tablespoon freshly grated gingerroot

1 tablespoon ground coriander

¼ tablespoon ground turmeric

1 cup water, divided

2 tablespoons olive oil

1 large serrano pepper, split into 4 slices

1 teaspoon cumin seed

1 large head cauliflower, cut into 1" pieces

1 cup Resistant Starch Potatoes (see recipe in this chapter), cut into small cubes

2 teaspoons salt, or to taste

3 tablespoons minced fresh cilantro, for garnish

1. In a small bowl, mix together the garlic, ginger, coriander, turmeric, and ½ cup water. (Wet spice mix).

2. In a large pot, heat the oil over medium heat and add the serrano peppers. Let them cook for 25–30 seconds. Immediately add the cumin seeds and cook until they begin to crack open.

3. Add the wet spice mix. Cook for 2–4 minutes.

4. Add the cauliflower and stir to coat the pieces with the spices. Add the remaining ½ cup water, cover, and cook for 10 minutes.

5. Add the potatoes and salt, stir, and cover for another 5 minutes. Remove the lid and keep stirring until the cauliflower is fully cooked. Approximately 3–5 minutes, Serve and garnish with fresh cilantro.

Chicken and Cauliflower Stir-Fry

Stir-fries are a fast and easy way to create a tasty meal. Serve this dish over Resistant Starch Brown Rice (see recipe in this chapter). You can also use whitefish instead of chicken or add other vegetables of your choice.

INGREDIENTS | SERVES 4

3 tablespoons olive oil

2 cloves garlic, minced

1 (3") piece gingerroot, sliced

1 pound skinless, boneless chicken breasts, cut into fajita-sized strips

Salt and freshly ground black pepper to taste

1 large head cauliflower, cut into bite-sized pieces

1 teaspoon ground cumin

1 tablespoon turmeric

½ teaspoon red pepper flakes

1 medium lemon, quartered

1. In a large pan or wok, heat the oil over high heat.

2. Add the garlic and sauté for 2 minutes.

3. Add the ginger and cook for 1 minute.

4. Add the chicken and season with salt and pepper. Cook for 5 minutes, stirring constantly.

5. Add the cauliflower, cumin, turmeric, red pepper flakes, and more salt and pepper.

6. Cook until the chicken is fully cooked and the cauliflower has cooked to desired doneness. Cook for 7–10 minutes.

7. Garnish with lemon wedges.

Chicken Breasts with Capers

Healthy and tangy, this dish is delicious over rice or salad. You can also add a ¼ cup of light coconut cream to this recipe for a creamy coconut flavor.

INGREDIENTS | SERVES 2

¼ cup olive oil
Juice of 2 medium lemons
1 clove garlic, minced
3 tablespoons capers, with brine
2 teaspoons salt
2 teaspoons freshly ground black pepper
2 (8-ounce) boneless, skinless chicken breasts

1. Preheat the oven to 350°F.

2. In a medium bowl, combine the oil, lemon juice, garlic, capers, salt, and pepper. Whisk to combine.

3. Place the chicken breast in a small baking dish. Pour the marinade on the chicken.

4. Bake uncovered for 35–40 minutes. Serve.

Halibut with Olives and Arugula

To turn this dish into a salad simply use the raw arugula and olives as a salad, place the cooked fish fillet on top, and dress it with olive oil, lemon, salt, and pepper.

INGREDIENTS | SERVES 2

3 tablespoons olive oil
2 (8-ounce) halibut fillets
Salt to taste
Freshly ground black pepper to taste
1 cup sliced kalamata olives
2 cups fresh arugula

1. In a large skillet, heat the oil over medium-high heat.

2. Season the fish with salt and pepper. Add the fish to the skillet and cook the fish for 4 minutes per side.

3. Remove the fish from the pan and set aside. Reduce the heat to medium.

4. Add the olives and arugula to the pan and season with salt and pepper. Cook for 4 minutes.

5. Pour this mixture on top of the fish fillets and serve.

Olive and Capers Pasta

If you love a refreshing vegetarian pasta for lunch, this dish is for you!
You can also replace the pasta with Resistant Starch Brown Rice (see recipe in this chapter).

INGREDIENTS | SERVES 2

¼ cup extra-virgin olive oil

Juice of 2 medium lemons

1 cup Resistant Starch Brown Rice Pasta (see recipe in this chapter)

1 cup diced kalamata olives

¼ cup capers

2 tablespoons finely chopped purple onion

¼ cup chopped fresh Italian parsley

Salt and freshly ground black pepper to taste

1. In a small bowl, combine the oil and lemon juice.

2. In a medium bowl, combine the pasta, olives, capers, onion, and parsley.

3. Pour the dressing over the pasta and toss.

4. Add salt and pepper to taste.

CHAPTER 12

Dinner

Rosemary and Sage Chicken
182

Moroccan-Inspired Sea Bass
183

Indian-Spiced Chicken Tenders
184

Herbes de Provence–Crusted
Halibut
185

Perfect and Tender Pot Roast
185

Seared Ahi Tuna Steaks
186

Pan-Seared Salmon with
Oregano
186

Hugo's Carne Asada–Style
Flank Steak
187

Spanish Lamb Steaks
188

Lemon Pepper Whitefish
188

Turmeric Rice and Chicken
189

Sizzling Grilled Lamb Chops
190

The Perfect Salmon Burgers
190

Casablanca Chicken Skewers
191

Chicken Fried Rice
192

Salmon Pockets
193

Creamy Spaghetti Squash
Vegetarian Pasta
194

Rosemary and Sage Chicken

Roasting a whole chicken is an easy way to make a great dinner for the family.

INGREDIENTS | SERVES 4

1 tablespoon ground sage

1½ tablespoons minced fresh rosemary
  or 1½ teaspoons dried rosemary

4 teaspoons sea salt

1 teaspoon garlic powder

3 teaspoons freshly ground black pepper

1 (5-pound) whole chicken

2 tablespoons olive oil

Cooking Chicken

When roasting chicken in the oven, always bake it breast side up. Bake the chicken at 375°F for 20 minutes per pound of chicken.

1. Preheat the oven to 375°F.

2. In a small bowl, combine the sage, rosemary, salt, garlic powder, and pepper.

3. Place the chicken in a large baking pan. Remove the giblets and discard, or reserve for another use.

4. Rub the chicken with olive oil. (This will help keep the chicken nice and crisp and also serve as glue for the spices.)

5. Evenly sprinkle the spice mix on the chicken.

6. Place the chicken in the oven and cook for 1 hour and 40 minutes. Or until internal temperature has reached 165°F.

7. Remove the chicken from the oven. Let rest for 10 minutes before carving.

Moroccan-Inspired Sea Bass

This marinade works great with any type of whitefish.
Use it with red snapper, sole, cod, halibut, or whatever you like!

INGREDIENTS | SERVES 2

1 tablespoon toasted cumin seed

3 cloves garlic, crushed

1 tablespoon chopped fresh Italian parsley

1 teaspoon sea salt

½ teaspoon freshly ground black pepper

1 tablespoon olive oil

3 tablespoons fresh lemon juice

1 pound Chilean sea bass, cut into 2 (8-ounce) fillets

1. Using a mortar and pestle, grind the toasted cumin seed with the garlic, parsley, salt, pepper, olive oil, and lemon juice.

2. Place the fish fillets in a medium baking pan and pour the spice paste on the fish, making sure that every piece is covered with the spices.

3. Cover with plastic wrap and marinate in the refrigerator for 1 hour.

4. Preheat the oven to 350°F.

5. Remove the plastic wrap from the pan and bake the fish for 20 minutes.

6. Remove the fish from the oven and serve over resistance starch rice or salad.

Indian-Spiced Chicken Tenders

If you like spicy food, you'll enjoy this delicious and juicy chicken dish.

INGREDIENTS | SERVES 4–6

1 cup light coconut milk

1 teaspoon ground turmeric

1 teaspoon garam masala

1 teaspoon ground coriander

1 teaspoon sea salt

1 teaspoon freshly ground black pepper

Pinch cayenne pepper

1 tablespoon olive oil

1 tablespoon lemon juice

2 pounds boneless, skinless chicken tenders

Garam Masala

This magnificent blend combines carda-
mom, cinnamon, cloves, cumin, black pepper, and coriander. It is a staple in many
Indian dishes.

1. In a medium bowl, combine the coconut milk, spices, oil, and lemon juice. Whisk them together.

2. Meanwhile, place the chicken tenders in an 8" square baking dish.

3. Pour the marinade over the chicken, making sure that every piece is covered with the mixture.

4. Cover with plastic wrap and refrigerate for 1 hour or overnight for more taste.

5. Preheat the oven to 350°F.

6. Bake the chicken for 40 minutes. Enjoy over resistant starch brown rice.

Herbes de Provence–Crusted Halibut

Be transported to the southeastern region of France with this decadent fish recipe. Halibut is lean fish, containing 50 percent less fat than salmon.

INGREDIENTS | SERVES 2

2 tablespoons olive oil

1 teaspoon sea salt

2 teaspoons freshly ground black pepper

2 tablespoons Herbes de Provence

1 pound halibut, cut into 2 (8-ounce) fillets

1. Preheat the oven to 350°F.

2. In a large skillet over medium-high heat, heat the oil.

3. Meanwhile, sprinkle the salt, pepper, and Herbes de Provence on the flesh side of the fish. Make sure the herbs evenly cover the fish; this will help create a nice crust.

4. Place the fish fillets flesh-side down in the skillet and cook for 5 minutes, until it has a nice brown crust.

5. Place the fillets skin side down in a medium baking dish. Place in the oven and bake for 4–5 minutes.

Perfect and Tender Pot Roast

Making pot roast is an easy way to create a large meal for the family. It is juicy, flavorful, and delicious.

INGREDIENTS | SERVES 6–8

3 tablespoons olive oil

1 (3–4 pound) chuck roast

Salt and freshly ground black pepper to taste

3 cups gluten-free beef stock

1½ teaspoons ground cumin

6 medium carrots peeled, cut into large chunks

4 celery stalks, cut into big chunks

4 medium shallots, cut in half

2 cloves garlic, crushed

2 bay leaves

3 sprigs rosemary

1. Heat a large pan over medium-high heat. Add the olive oil.

2. Season the roast generously with salt and pepper. Place the roast in the hot oil and sear it for about 5 minutes per side to create a nice brown crust.

3. Place the roast in a slow cooker.

4. To the slow cooker, add the stock, cumin, carrots, celery, shallots, garlic, bay leaves, rosemary, and more salt and pepper if needed.

5. Cover the slow cooker and cook for 3–4 hours at medium temperature until the roast is falling-apart tender.

Seared Ahi Tuna Steaks

Tuna is a wonderful fish that cooks fast and makes a delicious dinner over salad or rice.

INGREDIENTS | SERVES 2

2 (6-ounce) tuna steaks

2 teaspoons salt

2 teaspoons coarsely ground black pepper

4 teaspoons dried oregano

3 tablespoons olive oil

1 medium lemon, cut into 4 wedges

Tuna

The best way to eat tuna steaks is by searing them. The center is raw, but you still get a nice brown top. Cook for about 1½ minutes per side for rare; give it an extra minute for medium-rare.

1. Season the tuna steaks evenly with the salt, pepper, and oregano.

2. In a medium pan, heat the oil over medium heat.

3. Place the tuna steaks in the hot oil and sear for 1½ minutes on each side.

4. Make sure that every corner has been seared. This will give you a rare temperature. Cook for another minute on each side for medium-rare.

5. Serve immediately, and squeeze lemon juice (from wedges) on steaks.

Pan-Seared Salmon with Oregano

Salmon is a healthy fish high in omega-3 fatty acids.
Always eat wild when possible. Enjoy this dish over your favorite salad.

INGREDIENTS | SERVES 2

2 (8-ounce) fillets wild salmon

2 teaspoons salt

1 teaspoon freshly ground black pepper

1 tablespoon dried oregano

2 tablespoons olive oil

1 medium lemon, cut in half

Variation

If you'd like you can replace the dried oregano with dried basil. Another option is to combine oregano and basil. This combination works great!

1. Begin by placing the salmon fillets on a large plate.

2. Season the salmon fillets evenly with the salt, pepper, and oregano.

3. Heat the oil in a medium pan over medium heat.

4. Cook the salmon flesh side down first. Cook each side for 4 minutes.

5. Serve the salmon with the lemon on the side, squeeze on the lemon juice right before eating.

Hugo's Carne Asada–Style Flank Steak

Use this steak to make tacos on lettuce tortillas, or make a taco bowl with Resistant Starch Brown Rice (see recipe in Chapter 11).

INGREDIENTS | SERVES 6–8

1 cup orange juice

½ cup lemon juice

½ cup olive oil

½ cup Braggs Liquid Aminos

5 cloves garlic, crushed

1 large white onion, diced

2 tablespoons dried oregano

1 tablespoon chili powder

1 tablespoon paprika

1 tablespoon ground cumin

1½ teaspoons salt

1 tablespoon freshly ground black pepper

1 teaspoon red pepper flakes

2 cups finely chopped fresh cilantro

3 pounds flank steak

1. In a large bowl, combine the orange juice, lemon juice, olive oil, Braggs Liquid Aminos, garlic, onion, oregano, chili powder, paprika, cumin, salt, pepper, red pepper flakes, and cilantro. Whisk to incorporate all the ingredients.

2. Place the flank steak in a large baking pan.

3. Pour the marinade on the steak, making sure the entire steak is covered by the marinade. Let marinate in the refrigerator overnight, or for at least 5 hours.

4. Grill the meat over medium-high heat for 5–6 minutes on each side. This will make a nice medium-rare temperature.

Spanish Lamb Steaks

This marvelous recipe is great served as tapas at parties. If you'd like to serve this recipe at a party, cut the lamb into cubes before cooking. Use toothpicks to serve them on a big platter.

INGREDIENTS | SERVES 2

¼ cup orange juice

2½ tablespoons lemon juice

2 tablespoons lemon zest

3 teaspoons salt

1 tablespoon freshly ground black pepper

1 teaspoon ground cumin

1 teaspoon ground coriander

1 teaspoon chopped fresh thyme

2 cloves garlic, chopped finely

1 medium purple onion, chopped finely

½ cup plus 2 tablespoons olive oil, divided

2 pounds lamb leg, cut into 4 (8-ounce) steak-sized pieces

1. In a medium bowl, combine the orange juice, lemon juice, lemon zest, salt, pepper, cumin, coriander, thyme, garlic, onion and ½ cup olive oil. Whisk to incorporate all the ingredients.

2. Pour the marinade over the lamb steaks and let marinate in the refrigerator overnight, or for at least 5 hours.

3. In a large pan over medium-high heat, heat the 2 tablespoons olive oil.

4. Cook the lamb steaks for 4 minutes per side, or until they reach the desired doneness.

Lemon Pepper Whitefish

Use any whitefish for this recipe. Halibut or sea bass would both make excellent choices.

INGREDIENTS | SERVES 2

1 clove garlic, chopped into small pieces

2 teaspoons lemon pepper spice mix

1½ teaspoons sea salt

¼ teaspoon paprika

Pinch cayenne pepper

2 (8-ounce) halibut fillets

2 tablespoons olive oil

1. In a small bowl, combine the garlic, lemon pepper, salt, paprika, and cayenne pepper.

2. Rub the spice mix on the fish fillets. Place the fillets in a covered dish and let marinate in the fridge for 30 minutes.

3. In a medium skillet over medium heat, heat the oil.

4. Place the fish in the pan and cook for 3–4 minutes on each side.

5. Serve over rice or salad.

Grill It!

You can also grill this fish for a smoky flavor and beautiful grill marks. It would be perfect for a picnic day!

Turmeric Rice and Chicken

Healthy, flavorful, and moist, this is the perfect dish for a holiday meal.

INGREDIENTS | SERVES 2

2 tablespoons olive oil

1 pound boneless, skinless chicken breasts, cut into small cubes

Salt and freshly ground black pepper to taste

2 cups Resistant Starch Brown Rice (see recipe in Chapter 11)

1 cup gluten-free chicken stock

Pinch cayenne pepper

1 tablespoon ground turmeric

Variation

Blend the gluten-free chicken stock with a bunch of fresh cilantro, and add this juice to the rice. This makes a green rice with a wonderful cilantro flavor.

1. Heat the oil in a medium pan over medium heat.

2. Place the chicken in the hot oil and immediately season with salt and pepper.

3. Stir the chicken occasionally and cook for 8 minutes, or until the chicken is almost cooked.

4. Add the rice and stir.

5. Add the chicken stock, cayenne, and turmeric and stir.

6. Cover and cook until the chicken stock evaporates, stirring occasionally.

Sizzling Grilled Lamb Chops

Your family will be impressed with this dish. The grill marks and aroma will make your mouth water.

INGREDIENTS | SERVES 4

3 cloves garlic, crushed

1 tablespoon fresh rosemary leaves

1 teaspoon fresh thyme leaves

1 teaspoon ground cumin

¼ teaspoon paprika

3 tablespoons olive oil

Salt and freshly ground black pepper to taste

6–7 (4-ounces each) lamb chops

1. In a food processor blend the garlic, rosemary, thyme, cumin, paprika, olive oil, salt, and pepper. This will make a paste.

2. Rub the paste on the lamb chops. Cover the lamb chops and place in the refrigerator for 2 hours.

3. Heat the grill to high.

4. Place the lamb chops on the grill and cook for 3 minutes.

5. Flip the chops and grill for another 3 minutes. This will make a medium-rare chop; cook longer if desired.

The Perfect Salmon Burgers

This recipe brings salmon burgers to the next level: they are delicious and juicy. Serve these on a bed of mixed greens.

INGREDIENTS | SERVES 2

1 pound salmon, chopped into small pieces

1 clove garlic, chopped

1 small jalapeño pepper, seeded and chopped

2 teaspoons lemon pepper

1½ teaspoons salt

1 teaspoon freshly ground black pepper

2 tablespoons olive oil

1. In a medium bowl, combine the salmon, garlic, jalapeño, lemon pepper, salt, and pepper. Using your hands mix all the ingredients together. Form 2 equal patties.

2. Let the patties marinate in the fridge for 20–30 minutes.

3. In a large pan over medium heat, warm up the oil.

4. Cook the patties for 4–5 minutes on each side, or until cooked to desired doneness.

Casablanca Chicken Skewers

Be transported to the city of Casablanca with this marvelous recipe. Serve it on a bed of Resistant Starch Brown Rice (see recipe in Chapter 11). This recipe also works wonderfully with fish.

INGREDIENTS | SERVES 6

3½ teaspoons lemon pepper spice mix

1¼ teaspoons ground turmeric

1¼ teaspoons ground coriander

3 teaspoons paprika

2 teaspoons salt

1 teaspoon freshly ground black pepper

½ teaspoon ground cumin

¼ teaspoon cayenne pepper

2 pounds boneless, skinless chicken breasts, cut into 2" cubes

8 bamboo skewers soaked in water for 20 minutes

1. In a small bowl, combine the lemon pepper spice mix, turmeric, coriander, paprika, salt, pepper, cumin, and cayenne pepper.

2. Place the chicken in a large bowl.

3. Pour the spice mix on the chicken. Mix well to make sure every piece is covered by the spices.

4. Cover the bowl and refrigerate for at least 2 hours.

5. Make the skewers using the presoaked bamboo sticks. Thread approximately ¼-pound of chicken on each skewer.

6. Heat the grill on medium-high.

7. Grill the skewers for approximately 8 minutes per side, or until the chicken is fully cooked.

Chicken Fried Rice

Here are all the flavors that you love from the classic fried rice with a healthy approach. You can add your favorite vegetables to this recipe. Zucchini and carrots work great.

INGREDIENTS | SERVES 2

5 tablespoons olive oil, divided

3 large eggs

1 clove garlic, minced

1 tablespoon minced fresh gingerroot

2 cups Resistant Starch Brown Rice (see recipe in Chapter 11)

1 pound boneless, skinless chicken breasts, cut into small strips and cooked

½ purple onion, sliced

1 cup bean sprouts

3 tablespoons Braggs Liquid Aminos

½ cup chopped fresh cilantro

1. In a medium skillet over medium heat, warm 1 tablespoon oil. Add the eggs and scramble them in the pan. Set the scrambled eggs aside.

2. In a large pan over medium heat, heat the remaining 4 tablespoons olive oil.

3. Add the garlic and ginger, and cook for 1 minute.

4. Add the brown rice and cook for 2 minutes, stirring frequently.

5. Add the cooked chicken and stir to combine.

6. Add the onions and bean sprouts. Cook for 2 more minutes.

7. Add the scrambled eggs and stir.

8. Add the Braggs Liquid Aminos; this should create steam. Stir until the entire mixture is seasoned with the Bragg, about 2 minutes.

9. Add the cilantro and stir for 1 minute. Serve.

Salmon Pockets

This is a great technique to cook fish. You can put in all your veggies along with the fish and have a full dinner ready in less than 30 minutes.

INGREDIENTS | SERVES 2

2 tablespoons olive oil, divided

3 medium carrots peeled, cut in half lengthwise

3 medium parsnips peeled, cut in half lengthwise

2 (8-ounce) wild salmon fillets

Salt and freshly ground black pepper to taste

1 teaspoon ground turmeric

4 fresh basil leaves, julienned

1 medium lemon, sliced

Change the Fish

If you don't like salmon or prefer a leaner fish, try this recipe with sea bass or halibut.

1. Preheat the oven to 350°F.

2. Cut 2 squares of aluminum foil big enough to fully seal the pouches, approximately 8" long × 12" wide.

3. Begin by drizzling 1 tablespoon oil on the part of the foil where the vegetables will be placed.

4. Divide the carrots and parsnips into equal portions. Place the strips on the center of the foil sheets.

5. Place the salmon fillets on top of the carrot and parsnip strips. Drizzle the remaining olive oil on the salmon fillets. Season with salt, pepper, and turmeric.

6. Sprinkle the basil on the fillets, and place lemon slices on top.

7. Seal the pouches tightly, and bake for 30 minutes.

Creamy Spaghetti Squash Vegetarian Pasta

You won't believe this recipe is dairy-free. The creamy sauce makes everyone want to go for seconds.

INGREDIENTS | SERVES 4

1 medium spaghetti squash, cut in half lengthwise

2 tablespoons olive oil

1 clove garlic, minced

1 (14-ounce) can light coconut milk

½ (7-ounce) can full fat coconut milk

¼ cup drained capers

Juice of 3 medium lemons

1 tablespoon fresh chopped dill

Salt and freshly ground black pepper to taste

Make It with Chicken

Make it a chicken pasta by adding grilled chicken or pan-seared chicken to this dish.

1. Place the squash in a large pot and fill with plenty of water to cover the entire squash.

2. Boil for 35 minutes or until the squash is fully cooked. Using a fork, remove the squash meat and set aside.

3. In a large pan, heat the oil over medium heat. Add the garlic and cook for 1 minute.

4. Add the coconut milks, capers, lemon juice, dill, salt, and pepper. Stir the sauce for 2 minutes or until it begins to bubble.

5. Add the squash to the sauce and toss with the heat still on. Serve hot.

CHAPTER 13

Sauces and Marinades

Turmeric Mayonnaise
196

Lemon-Ginger Salad Dressing
196

Hugo's Homemade
Chicken Stock
197

Indian-Inspired Chicken
Marinade
198

Cilantro Lime Marinade
198

South of the Border Aioli
199

Lamb Marinade
199

Argentinean Steak Chimichurri
200

Mint Chutney
200

Pumpkin Spice Applesauce
201

Pure and Natural
Cranberry Sauce
202

Killer Jalapeño Relish
202

Kalamata Olive Spread
203

Asian Marinade
203

Ceviche Marinade
(*Leche de Tigre*)
204

Turmeric Mayonnaise

Add a touch of flavor and anti-inflammatory properties to your food with this recipe.

INGREDIENTS | MAKES ABOUT 2 CUPS

2 large egg yolks

¼ cup lemon juice

Salt to taste

1 tablespoon ground turmeric

1½ cups extra-virgin olive oil

Raw Eggs

Mayonnaise contains raw eggs. Because of this you should always use fresh eggs from a reliable source.

1. In a food processor, combine the egg yolks, lemon juice, salt, and turmeric.

2. Turn the machine on low speed and mix for 30 seconds, just enough to combine the ingredients.

3. With the food processor still running, slowly drizzle in the oil. The mixture will begin to thicken. Continue drizzling until you run out of oil.

4. If you find your mayonnaise is too watery, add a little more oil.

5. Store in the refrigerator for up to 1 week.

Lemon-Ginger Salad Dressing

This dressing is perfect on top of mixed greens or raw zucchini salad.

INGREDIENTS | MAKES ABOUT 1 CUP

¼ cup lemon juice

½ cup extra-virgin olive oil

2 tablespoons minced gingerroot

¼ teaspoon salt

¼ teaspoon freshly ground black pepper

Blend It

If you're in a rush and want to make this dressing faster, simply throw all the ingredients in a blender.

1. In a medium bowl, whisk together all the ingredients until fully incorporated.

2. Let the dressing rest for 20 minutes to allow the flavors of the ginger to come out.

3. Whisk right before serving.

Hugo's Homemade Chicken Stock

Having chicken stock available in the fridge is always helpful. Use to make rice, soups, and stews.

INGREDIENTS | MAKES ABOUT 6 CUPS

1 (5-pound) whole chicken

2 large carrots peeled, cut into big chucks

2 large stalks celery

1 large yellow onion, quartered

1 medium green bell pepper, quartered

1 clove garlic, mashed

1 large onion, quartered

3 sprigs thyme

2 bay leaves

7 whole peppercorns

2 sprigs rosemary

8 cups water

Salt It at the End

With broth it's better to make it unsalted. When the broth is done you may salt it, or just salt what you need.

1. Cut the chicken into quarters. Place the chicken in a large stockpot.

2. Add the vegetables and herbs.

3. Add the water, and bring to a boil over medium-high heat. Boil for 3 minutes.

4. Reduce the heat to low, and let simmer for 2 hours.

5. Turn off the heat and let cool for 15 minutes before straining.

6. Strain the stock, saving the chicken for other recipes and discarding the other solids.

7. Salt the stock before consuming.

Indian-Inspired Chicken Marinade

This recipe is rich in flavor and healthy for your family. You can use this marinade on chicken or whitefish.

INGREDIENTS | MAKES ABOUT 2 CUPS

1½ cups light coconut cream
¼ cup lemon juice
¼ cup extra-virgin olive oil
1 tablespoon garam masala
2 tablespoons ground turmeric
2 tablespoons grated fresh gingerroot
2 tablespoons ground coriander
2 cloves garlic, mashed
2 teaspoons ground cumin
¼ teaspoon cayenne pepper
½ cup chopped fresh cilantro
2 teaspoons salt
2 teaspoons freshly ground black pepper

1. In a blender combine all the ingredients. Blend until all the ingredients are incorporated.

2. Refrigerate immediately. It will keep in the fridge for up to 1 week.

3. Marinate your fish or chicken in this mixture for at least 2 hours before cooking.

Cilantro Lime Marinade

Use this recipe when you are craving something tangy and fresh.
This marinade is perfect for chicken, but works well with beef too.

INGREDIENTS | MAKES 2 CUPS

1 cup fresh lemon juice
¼ cup extra-virgin olive oil
2 bunches fresh cilantro
1 medium jalapeño pepper, seeded
¾ cup water
2 teaspoons salt
2 teaspoons freshly ground black pepper
2 cloves garlic, mashed
1 medium white onion, quartered

1. Put all the ingredients in a blender. Blend until all the ingredients are incorporated.

2. Refrigerate. It will keep in the fridge for up to 1 week.

3. Marinate your chicken, or protein of choice, in this mixture for at least 2 hours before cooking.

South of the Border Aioli

This is a delicious sauce to enjoy with any dish. Put it on your rice, cooked chicken, beef, or fish.

INGREDIENTS | MAKES 1¼ CUPS

1 cup homemade mayonnaise
1 large jalapeño
½ cup chopped fresh cilantro
1 tablespoon fresh lemon juice
2 teaspoons salt
2 teaspoons freshly ground black pepper

1. Put all ingredients in a blender. Blend until all the ingredients are incorporated.

2. The aioli should be smooth and slightly green in color.

3. Store in a covered container in the refrigerator. Keeps for 1 week.

Too Hot for You?

If you find this aioli to be too hot for your taste buds, simply remove the seeds and veins from the jalapeño. Or if you desire more heat, add more jalapeño.

Lamb Marinade

This Greek-style marinade works great on lamb chops, or lamb loin cooked over open fire. If you don't have access to fresh oregano, try using dried oregano or fresh or dried rosemary.

INGREDIENTS | MAKES 1 CUP

1 cup extra-virgin olive oil
2 tablespoons fresh lemon juice
1 cup chopped fresh oregano, or ½ cup dried
1½ teaspoons salt
1½ teaspoons freshly ground black pepper
1 teaspoon ground cumin
3 cloves garlic, finely chopped

1. In a large bowl, whisk together all the ingredients.

2. Immediately pour over lamb, and let marinate in the refrigerator for 2 hours or overnight for more flavor.

Argentinean Steak Chimichurri

Chimichurri is a delicious blend of herbs and garlic in a base of oil. It is used as a topping for grilled steaks, but is delicious with any grilled protein.

INGREDIENTS | MAKES 2 CUPS

1¾ cups finely chopped fresh Italian parsley

3 cloves garlic, minced

2 medium shallots, minced

2 tablespoons chopped fresh oregano

¼ cup fresh lemon juice

1 cup extra-virgin olive oil

½ teaspoon red pepper flakes

1¼ teaspoons salt, or more to taste

1 teaspoon freshly ground black pepper

1. In a food processor add all the ingredients. Blend the ingredients just enough to get a chunky texture but not a paste. The easiest way to achieve this is by pulsing the ingredients.

2. You may also chop all the ingredients finely, and then mix them together in a bowl.

Mint Chutney

*Enjoy this chutney with your favorite lamb or chicken dish.
It is the perfect complement to your East Asian recipe.*

INGREDIENTS | MAKES 1½ CUPS

2 cups fresh mint leaves

1 bunch fresh cilantro

1 serrano pepper

1½ tablespoons lemon juice

½ teaspoon salt, or more to taste

½" piece fresh gingerroot, peeled

5 tablespoons water

1. Place all the ingredients in a food processor.

2. Blend the ingredients, adding water as needed. You want to achieve a fine paste.

3. Taste it for salt and add more if desired.

4. If you desire more heat, this is the time to add another serrano pepper and blend.

Variations

If you enjoy the flavor of onion, try adding 1 medium onion to this recipe. In addition to giving it more flavor, the onion will add more texture to this chutney.

Pumpkin Spice Applesauce

This makes the perfect snack for the holidays. Enjoy with breakfast, have it as dessert, or simply eat it as a snack!

INGREDIENTS | MAKES 2 CUPS

8 Gala apples, peeled, cored, and cut into quarters

2 teaspoons ground cinnamon

2 tablespoons pumpkin pie spice mix

½ teaspoon ground ginger

¼ teaspoon salt

Creamy Variation

Looking for a creamier version of this recipe? Simply, add 1½ tablespoons coconut oil to achieve a creamier and richer texture. Coconut oil crystallizes at cold temperatures, so the sauce may harden a little when cold.

1. Preheat the oven to 350°F.

2. Place the apples in a large baking pan.

3. Add the spices and salt to the apples. Mix the apples with your hands, making sure that every piece is covered by the seasonings.

4. Bake the apples for 45 minutes, until soft.

5. Remove from the oven and let cool for 8–10 minutes.

6. Transfer to a blender. Blend at medium speed until you have a smooth texture.

Pure and Natural Cranberry Sauce

Want to cut back on the sugars during the holidays? This is the recipe for you!

INGREDIENTS | MAKES 2 CUPS

4 cups fresh cranberries
3 cups freshly squeezed orange juice
1 tablespoon orange zest
2 tablespoons freshly grated gingerroot
¼ teaspoon salt

Add a Touch of Honey

If you don't have any problems with honey, add 1 tablespoon of raw honey to this recipe. The honey will add a touch of sweetness, while still maintaining the tartness of the cranberries.

1. Place all the ingredients in a medium saucepan. Cook over high heat until the mixture boils.

2. Reduce heat and simmer uncovered for 25–30 minutes, or until the cranberries start to dissolve.

3. Once the cranberries are nice and soft, mash them with a potato masher or fork.

4. Place in the fridge for 30 minutes. Serve cold.

Killer Jalapeño Relish

Add this relish to pretty much anything that you want to turn into a killer hot plate. This recipe is made out of pure jalapeño heat!

INGREDIENTS | MAKES 1 CUP

12 large jalapeños
1 tablespoon fresh lemon juice
1 teaspoon salt, or more to taste

Pour Over Tacos!

This sauce is delicious over your homemade Tex-Mex dishes. Make your favorite tacos at home and use this relish instead of the salsa. Remember that a little goes a long way.

1. Preheat the oven to 375°F.

2. Wash all the jalapeño peppers. Place in a baking pan and roast the jalapeños for 30 minutes.

3. Transfer the roasted jalapeños to a food processor.

4. Add the lemon juice and salt. Blend until you a have a chunky relish texture.

5. Place the relish in an airtight container and refrigerate until the relish is cold.

6. Taste the relish and add more salt if needed.

Kalamata Olive Spread

This is delicious as a dip, or use it on top of grilled chicken or steak. You can also replace half the kalamata olives for half green olives to achieve a different flavor profile and color.

INGREDIENTS | SERVES 4

2 cloves garlic

½ cup fresh Italian parsley leaves

2 tablespoons extra-virgin olive oil

Juice of 2 medium lemons

1 cup pitted kalamata olives

Salt and freshly ground black pepper to taste

1. To a food processor, add the garlic, parsley, olive oil, and lemon juice. Pulse to mince.

2. Add the olives and blend until you get a creamy-coarse texture.

3. Add salt and pepper to taste. Eat immediately or refrigerate for up to 1 week.

Asian Marinade

Use this marinade for fish or beef. It is sweet and salty with a little ginger kick. You can also add 1 medium purple onion to this marinade for more flavor.

INGREDIENTS | SERVES 2

1 cup Braggs Liquid Aminos

2 cloves garlic

4 tablespoons extra-virgin olive oil

1 (3") piece fresh gingerroot

2 tablespoons raw honey

1. Add all the ingredients to a food processor or blender. Blend on high for 3 minutes.

2. Use it immediately or keep in the fridge for up to 1 week.

Ceviche Marinade (*Leche de Tigre*)

This is the base to make a fresh Peruvian-style ceviche.
Some people like to drink this as a shot called leche de tigre (tiger's milk).

INGREDIENTS | SERVES 1

1 cup freshly squeezed lemon juice

2 cloves garlic

1 medium or small purple onion, quartered

6 ounces whitefish fillet

1" piece fresh gingerroot

2 teaspoons salt

1 teaspoon freshly ground black pepper

10 ice cubes

1. In a blender add the lemon juice, garlic, onion, fish fillet, and ginger. Blend on medium speed.

2. Add the salt, pepper, and 4 ice cubes. Blend on high until the ice is crushed.

3. Add a few more ice cubes at a time. Blend until you have a smoothie-like texture.

4. Use immediately.

To Make the Ceviche

To make ceviche with this sauce, simply cut 2 pounds of sea bass into cubes, pour the marinade over the fish, and stir. Let the fish marinate for at least 5 minutes, or longer if you like your fish a little more cooked by the lemon juice. Garnish with cilantro and boiled sweet potato.

CHAPTER 14

Soups and Stews

Carrot Turmeric Soup
206

Beet Soup
207

Coconut Cream of Broccoli Soup
208

Roasted Cauliflower and
Turmeric Soup
209

Butternut Squash Soup
210

Beef with Butternut Squash Stew
211

Hugo's Chicken *Albóndiga* Soup
212

Whitefish Soup
213

Russian Salmon Soup
214

Refreshing Avocado Soup
215

Silky Butternut Squash Soup
with Coconut Cream
216

Tom Kha Gai Soup
(Thai Coconut Chicken Soup)
217

Vegetable and Egg Soup
218

Parsnip and Turmeric Soup
219

Cucumber Mint Soup
220

Carrot Turmeric Soup

Turmeric contains curcumin, a wonderful and natural anti-inflammatory.

INGREDIENTS | SERVES 8–10 (1 CUP EACH)

1 tablespoon olive oil

1 clove garlic

1 tablespoon coconut oil

2 small shallots, peeled and cut into quarters

48 ounces gluten-free chicken stock

10 large carrots peeled, cut into 1" cubes

¼ cup grated fresh turmeric root

2 tablespoons grated fresh gingerroot

Salt and freshly ground black pepper to taste

¼ cup chopped parsley for garnish

Make It Creamy!

Add 1 cup light coconut cream from a can to make this soup a creamy dairy-free soup.

1. In a large pot (6-quart or bigger), heat the olive oil on medium-low. Add the garlic, coconut oil, and shallots, stirring until the shallots become translucent. This takes approximately 5 minutes.

2. Add the stock, carrots, turmeric, and ginger. Cover and bring to a boil.

3. Reduce the heat to low and let simmer until the carrots are tender and fully cooked (easily pierced with a fork). This process takes 10–15 minutes.

4. Remove from the heat and let cool for 15 minutes. Transfer to a blender.

5. Blend in batches, and transfer the blended soup back to the pot. Add salt and pepper to taste, and bring to a boil over medium heat. (This is the time to add the coconut cream if desired.)

6. Garnish with parsley.

Beet Soup

Beets contain betanin and vulgaxanthin, which have been shown to provide anti-inflammatory and detoxification support.

INGREDIENTS | SERVES 8

3 tablespoons coconut oil

2 small white onions, peeled and cut into quarters

48 ounces gluten-free vegetable stock

2 tablespoons grated fresh gingerroot

6–8 large beets, peeled and quartered

Salt and freshly ground black pepper to taste

1 tablespoon dill

Try It with Yellow Beets

Replace the red beets with yellow beets to make this soup into a fun yellow treat!

1. In a large pot (6-quart or bigger), heat the coconut oil over medium-low heat. Add the onions and cook, stirring until the onions become translucent, about 5 minutes.

2. Add the vegetable stock, ginger, and beets. Cover and bring to a boil.

3. Reduce the heat to low and let simmer until the beets are tender and fully cooked, about 15–20 minutes.

4. Remove from the heat and let cool for 15 minutes. Transfer to a blender.

5. Blend in batches, then transfer the puréed soup back to the pot and add salt and pepper to taste. Bring to a boil over medium heat.

6. Garnish with dill.

Coconut Cream of Broccoli Soup

This creamy dairy-free variation is a great way to get kids to eat their vegetables.

INGREDIENTS | SERVES 8

2 tablespoons olive oil

1 tablespoon coconut oil

1 medium white onion, chopped

1 clove garlic, chopped

2 medium russet potatoes, peeled and cut into quarters

8 cups finely chopped broccoli florets and stems

10 cups gluten-free chicken stock

1½ (14-ounce) cans light coconut milk, total of 21 ounces

Salt and freshly ground black pepper to taste

Natural Thickener

The russet potatoes in this recipe serve as a natural thickening agent to your soup, replacing any gluten base.

1. In a large pot over medium heat, warm up the olive and coconut oils.

2. Add the onion and garlic and cook until translucent approximately 5 minutes.

3. Add the potatoes, broccoli, and chicken stock and bring to a boil.

4. Reduce heat to low and let simmer until the broccoli and potatoes are fully cooked. This takes approximately 10 minutes.

5. Remove from heat and let cool for 15 minutes. Transfer to a blender and blend in batches.

6. Return to the pot, add the coconut milk and salt and pepper to taste, and bring to a boil over medium heat. Serve warm.

Roasted Cauliflower and Turmeric Soup

Did you know that cauliflower can be found in a variety of colors?
This magnificent vegetable can be found in white, orange, green, and purple.

INGREDIENTS | SERVES 8–10

2 large heads cauliflower, chopped into
   1" florets
1 medium white onion, chopped
1 clove garlic, chopped
3 tablespoons olive oil
4 cups gluten-free chicken stock
1 large russet potato, peeled and cut
   into quarters
1 tablespoon Herbes de Provence
2 cups light coconut milk
1 tablespoon ground turmeric
Salt and freshly ground black pepper to
   taste

Not All Cauliflowers Are Built the Same

Different color cauliflowers contain different nutritional properties. Use yellow cauliflower for more vitamin A and the purple variety for more antioxidants.

1. Preheat the oven to 425°F.

2. In a large baking pan, combine the cauliflower, onion, and garlic.

3. Drizzle the olive oil on top of the cauliflower mixture and toss to make sure all the pieces are covered in oil.

4. Bake for 25–30 minutes or until golden brown.

5. Transfer the contents to a large stockpot and add the chicken stock, potatoes, and Herbes de Provence.

6. Bring to a boil, then reduce to a simmer over medium heat and cook for 20 minutes or until the potatoes and cauliflower are soft and tender.

7. Remove from heat and let cool for 15 minutes. Transfer to a blender and blend in batches.

8. Return the mixture to the pot. Add the coconut milk, turmeric, and salt and pepper to taste. Bring to a boil over medium heat. Eat hot!

Butternut Squash Soup

Enjoy the silky and velvety texture of butternut squash with this wonderful soup. You can also try adding ½ cup coconut cream to this recipe to achieve a richer and creamier texture.

INGREDIENTS | SERVES 4–6

3 tablespoons olive oil

1 medium white onion, chopped

1 large butternut squash (about 3 pounds), cut into square chunks

6 cups gluten-free chicken stock

1 tablespoon ground turmeric

1½ teaspoons grated fresh nutmeg

Salt and freshly ground black pepper to taste

1. In a large soup pot over medium heat, heat the olive oil.

2. Add the onion and cook for 5 minutes, until translucent.

3. Add the squash and stir for 1 minute.

4. Add the chicken stock and cook over medium heat until the squash is cooked and tender, about 20 minutes.

5. Once the squash is cooked, place the cooked chunks in a blender. Add a little stock to make it easier to blend. Purée the squash.

6. Add the squash to the stock. Add the turmeric and nutmeg. Stir to combine the spices.

7. Add salt and pepper to taste. Serve immediately.

Beef with Butternut Squash Stew

Enjoy this creamy creation on a cold winter night. It is the perfect way to satisfy your pallet and tummy. This recipe also works great with lamb.

INGREDIENTS | SERVES 4

2 tablespoons olive oil

1 clove garlic, minced

2 pounds stew beef

Salt and freshly ground black pepper to taste

8 cups water or gluten-free beef stock, divided

1 bay leaf

1½ pounds butternut squash peeled, and cubed

1 tablespoon ground turmeric

1. In a large stockpot over medium heat, heat the oil.

2. Add the garlic and cook for 1 minute.

3. Add the beef, season it with salt and pepper, and stir occasionally until brown. This takes approximately 7–10 minutes.

4. Add 6 cups of water or beef stock and the bay leaf.

5. Cover and simmer on medium-low heat until the beef is tender, about 45 minutes.

6. Meanwhile, in a separate pot bring 2 cups water to a boil.

7. Add the squash to the water and cook for 20 minutes, until tender.

8. Place the cooked squash in a blender and process until smooth.

9. Add the puréed butternut squash to the cooked stew meat mixture, and stir to combine.

10. Add the turmeric and salt and pepper to taste. Remove bay leaf. Serve immediately.

Hugo's Chicken *Albóndiga* Soup

This is a healthier version of the Mexican classic. This recipe uses lean chicken instead of beef.

INGREDIENTS | SERVES 4

6½ cups of water

2 pounds ground chicken

2 teaspoons salt

1 teaspoon freshly ground black pepper

1 teaspoon ground sage

¼ teaspoon ground cumin

1 teaspoon ground turmeric

½ cup shredded carrots

1 cup Resistant Starch Brown Rice (see recipe in Chapter 11)

1 cup peeled and chopped carrots

1 cup chopped celery

½ bunch fresh cilantro springs

1. Bring water to a boil over medium heat.

2. While waiting for the water to boil, combine the chicken, spices, shredded carrots, and brown rice in a medium bowl. Mix well using your hands.

3. Make small 2" balls and add them directly to the water.

4. Add the chopped carrots and celery.

5. Cook for about 35 minutes, until the chicken balls are fully cooked.

6. Add more salt and pepper to taste if desired.

7. Add the cilantro sprigs to the soup, and turn off the heat. Your soup is now ready to be served.

Whitefish Soup

This soup is a staple in most coastal cities along the Andalusia region of Spain. If you can't find fish stock, simply replace it with chicken stock. The flavors vary, but you'll still get a delicious soup!

INGREDIENTS | SERVES 4

2 tablespoons olive oil

1 medium white onion, chopped

1 clove garlic, smashed

1 large carrot, peeled and diced

1 large celery stalk, diced

6 cups gluten-free fish stock

2 pounds whitefish, cubed

Salt and freshly ground black pepper to taste

1 medium lemon, cut into 4 wedges

1. In a medium pot over medium heat, heat the oil.

2. Add the onion, garlic, carrot, and celery. Cook for 5 minutes, until the onion is translucent.

3. Add the fish stock and bring to a boil.

4. Reduce heat and simmer for 5 minutes.

5. Add the fish. Cook for another 5 minutes, until the fish is fully cooked.

6. Add salt and pepper to taste. Serve hot with a lemon wedge.

Russian Salmon Soup

This is a variation to the Russian ukha, a soup made of salmon heads and tails.

INGREDIENTS | SERVES 4

4 tablespoons olive oil

1 medium yellow onion, chopped

3 small carrots, peeled and chopped

1 small celery root, chopped

1 small parsley root, chopped

6 cups gluten-free fish stock

5 whole peppercorns

2 bay leaves

1½ teaspoons red pepper flakes

3 pounds wild salmon, skin removed, cut into small cubes

Salt and freshly ground black pepper to taste

Sliced green onions, for garnish

1 medium lemon, cut into wedges

1. In a medium stockpot over medium heat, heat the oil.

2. Add the onion and root vegetables. Sauté for 5 minutes.

3. Add the fish stock, peppercorns, bay leaves, and red pepper flakes. Bring to a boil.

4. Reduce heat and simmer for 5 more minutes.

5. Add the salmon and cook for 7–10 minutes or until the salmon is cooked.

6. Remove the peppercorns and bay leaves, and add salt and pepper to taste.

7. Serve hot, and garnish with the green onions and lemon wedges.

A Pinch of Turmeric

Add turmeric to this recipe for color. Turmeric is an excellent anti-inflammatory and works great with soups.

Refreshing Avocado Soup

Enjoy this soup as an appetizer to any meal, or add some protein to make it a complete meal. You can also give this soup a creamy touch by adding ¼ cup light coconut milk.

INGREDIENTS | SERVES 2

2 large ripe avocados, peeled

1 teaspoon fresh lemon juice

1 medium cucumber

¾ cup gluten-free chicken stock

1 medium jalapeño pepper, seeded

5 sprigs fresh cilantro

Salt and freshly ground black pepper to taste

1. Place all the ingredients in a food processor. Blend until you have a creamy soup.

2. Taste the soup for salt. Add more if needed.

3. If the soup is too watery, add more avocado, or if the soup is too thick, add more chicken stock.

4. Serve cold.

Silky Butternut Squash Soup with Coconut Cream

If you love thick and creamy soups, you'll love this combination of butternut and coconut cream.

INGREDIENTS | SERVES 2

2 cups cubed butternut squash

2 tablespoons olive oil

1 (2") piece fresh gingerroot, sliced

1 large yellow onion, chopped

3 cups gluten-free chicken stock

2 teaspoons ground turmeric

7 ounces full fat coconut cream (milk)

Salt and freshly ground black pepper to taste

Sliced green onions, for garnish

Rich in Vitamin A

Butternut squash is full of vitamin A. This vitamin is known to keep your eyes healthy.

1. Preheat the oven to 375°F.

2. In a medium baking pan, combine the butternut squash, oil, ginger, and onion. Toss well to make sure that all the ingredients have been coated with the oil.

3. Bake for 50–60 minutes, until the butternut squash is tender.

4. Remove from the oven and let it rest for 15 minutes. Transfer the baked ingredients to a blender.

5. Add the chicken stock and turmeric. Blend until you have a creamy mixture.

6. Transfer to a medium pot and cook over medium heat for 5 minutes, or until it begins to boil.

7. Add coconut cream, salt and pepper to taste.

8. Serve warm and garnish with green onions.

Tom Kha Gai Soup (Thai Coconut Chicken Soup)

Here is a delicious spicy and creamy soup with a base of coconut milk and gluten-free chicken stock.

INGREDIENTS | SERVES 4–6

3½ cups gluten-free chicken stock

2½ cups gluten-free fish stock

1 clove garlic, smashed

5 small red shallots, diced

3 stalks fresh lemongrass, chopped white part only

2 pounds boneless, skinless chicken breasts, diced into small pieces

3" piece fresh gingerroot, sliced

Zest of 1 medium lime

½ teaspoon salt, or more to taste

1¾ cups button mushrooms

1 medium serrano pepper with seeds

1 medium serrano pepper, seeded

Juice of 7 medium limes

2 (14-ounce) cans light coconut milk

4–6 sprigs fresh cilantro

Fish Sauce

The traditional soup uses fish sauce, which is fermented. This recipe replaces that with fish stock, as fermented products may promote inflammation.

1. In a large soup pot over medium heat, combine the chicken stock, fish stock, garlic, shallots, and lemongrass. Let simmer for 15 minutes.

2. Strain the stock, and return to the pot.

3. Add the chicken, ginger, lime zest, salt, and mushrooms and simmer for another 15 minutes or until the chicken is cooked.

4. Add the serrano peppers and lime juice. Simmer for 3 minutes.

5. Add the coconut milk, and stir to combine. Simmer for 10 more minutes.

6. Serve hot, and add cilantro sprigs to each serving. Add more salt if needed.

Vegetable and Egg Soup

In this recipe the egg serves as the main source of protein. Feel free to add your favorite vegetables to this soup. If you're adding potatoes, make sure to use resistant starch potatoes.

INGREDIENTS | SERVES 4

5 cups gluten-free chicken stock

3 large carrots, peeled and diced

3 large stalks celery, diced

1 cup fresh spinach

2 medium zucchini, cut into big chunks

4 large eggs

Salt and freshly ground black pepper to taste

Sliced green onion, for garnish

1. In a large pot combine the chicken stock, carrots, and celery. Bring to a boil over medium heat. Cook for 10 minutes.

2. Add the spinach and zucchini and bring to a boil. Boil for 3 minutes.

3. While the soup is boiling, crack the eggs and add one at a time.

4. Cook for 5–7 minutes or until the eggs are hard-boiled.

5. Add salt and pepper to taste.

6. Serve the soup, adding one whole cooked egg to each bowl. Garnish with green onions.

Parsnip and Turmeric Soup

Parsnip has a distinct sweet taste that will be soothing to your palate.
The touch of fresh turmeric adds color and wonderful anti-inflammatory properties.

INGREDIENTS | SERVES 4–6

3 tablespoons coconut oil

1 large white onion, chopped

3 large stalks celery, chopped

1 clove garlic, chopped

Salt and freshly ground black pepper to taste

10 cups gluten-free chicken stock

1 bay leaf

2 (3") pieces fresh turmeric root, diced

3½ pounds parsnips, peeled and diced

½ cup light coconut milk

Chopped chives, for garnish

Thickening Agent

If you wish to thicken this soup, use 1 tablespoon of unmodified potato starch, which is considered a resistant starch.

1. In a large stock pot over medium heat, melt the coconut oil.

2. Add the onion, celery, and garlic. Season with salt and pepper. Cook until translucent. About 5 minutes.

3. Add the chicken stock, bay leaf, turmeric root, and parsnips.

4. Bring to a boil, then immediately reduce the heat and simmer for 1 hour or until the parsnips are soft.

5. Remove from heat and let cool for 10 minutes. Remove the bay leaf.

6. Transfer to a blender and blend in batches until smooth. Return to the pot and cook over medium heat.

7. Add the coconut milk. Add more salt and pepper to taste.

8. Garnish with chives, and serve warm.

Cucumber Mint Soup

This is the perfect soup to serve as an appetizer on a hot summer day.

INGREDIENTS | SERVES 2

12 large cucumbers, peeled

1 medium avocado, pit removed

Juice of 1 lemon

1 cup fresh mint

Salt and freshly ground black pepper to taste

Add More Texture

If you desire more texture, cut one cucumber into small chucks and add to the soup as garnish.

1. Place the cucumbers, avocado, lemon juice, and mint in a blender or food processor. Blend until creamy and smooth.

2. Add salt and pepper to taste and blend again.

3. Serve cold, and add a few mint leaves for garnish.

CHAPTER 15

Salads

Cucumber and Green
Bean Salad
222

Chicken and Brown Rice Salad
223

Chicken Salad with Apples
and Grapes
224

Root Slaw Salad
225

Mint and Watermelon Salad
225

Ginger Turmeric Potato Salad
226

Spiced Egg Salad
227

Ensalada de Jicama
(Jicama Salad)
228

Creamy Salmon Salad
229

Yellow Mayonnaise Beet Slaw
230

Mango and Jicama Salad
230

Roasted Beet Salad
231

Berry-Nutritious
Antioxidant Salad
232

Spiced Apples and Bananas
Dessert Salad
232

Asparagus Salad
233

Classic Coleslaw
233

Endive and Heart of Palm Salad
234

Blood Orange and
Arugula Salad
234

Cucumber and Green Bean Salad

Enjoy this salad with grilled chicken, fish, or simply eat it just the way it is.
Feel free to add a pinch of cayenne pepper for heat.

INGREDIENTS | SERVES 4

2 pounds green beans, ends removed

4 medium cucumbers, peeled and chopped into 1" chunks

1 tablespoon extra-virgin olive oil

Juice of 3 lemons

Salt and freshly ground black pepper to taste

1. Bring water to a boil in a medium pot and cook the green beans for 5 minutes. You may steam them if you wish.

2. Remove from heat, strain the green beans, and set aside.

3. In a large salad bowl, combine the green beans and cucumber chunks.

4. Add the olive oil and lemon juice. Do not add the dressing ingredients if you're not going to eat immediately.

5. Toss the salad to make sure that every green bean and cucumber is coated with oil and lemon.

6. Season with salt and pepper. Serve immediately.

Chicken and Brown Rice Salad

This is a cold salad prepared with Resistant Starch Brown Rice.
It is a complete meal that will satisfy your hunger.

INGREDIENTS | SERVES 2

1 pound chicken breast

¼ cup fresh lemon juice

¼ cup extra-virgin olive oil

1 tablespoon ground turmeric

Salt and freshly ground black pepper to taste

2 cups Resistant Starch Brown Rice (see recipe in Chapter 11)

1 cup diced cremini mushrooms

2 medium stalks celery, diced

2 medium carrots, peeled and diced

¼ cup chopped fresh Italian parsley

How to Clean Mushrooms

Mushrooms act as sponges, so it is best not to wash them in water. The best way to clean them is by using a wet paper towel to scrub the surface of the mushrooms.

1. In a medium pot, bring enough salted water to a boil to cook the chicken. Boil the chicken for 20–25 minutes. Remove the chicken from the heat and let cool. Shred the chicken and set aside.

2. Meanwhile, in a small bowl make the dressing: whisk together the lemon juice, olive oil, turmeric, salt, and pepper.

3. In a medium salad bowl, combine the rice, chicken, mushrooms, vegetables, and parsley.

4. Pour the dressing on the salad mixture and toss. Check for salt and pepper and add more if desired.

5. Let it sit for 5 minutes before serving.

Chicken Salad with Apples and Grapes

*This salad is a mouth-watering sweet and savory combination
of crispy apples, sweet grapes, and chicken.*

INGREDIENTS | SERVES 4

1 pound boneless, skinless chicken breasts, cut into 1"cubes

1 Gala apple, cored and cut into 1" chunks

2 medium stalks celery, diced

1 cup halved red grapes

½ cup homemade mayonnaise

1 teaspoon salt

1½ teaspoons freshly ground black pepper

Add Some Crunch

If you don't have any problems with nuts, try adding some almonds or walnuts to this recipe. This will add more texture to your salad.

1. In a medium pot, bring enough salted water to a boil to cook the chicken. Boil the chicken for 20–25 minutes. Remove the chicken from the heat and let cool.

2. In a large bowl combine the apples, celery, grapes, and cooled chicken.

3. Add the mayonnaise and mix to combine.

4. Add salt and pepper to taste and combine again.

5. Place in the fridge for at least 15 minutes before serving.

6. Serve on a bed of iceberg lettuce if desired.

Root Slaw Salad

This recipe combines three wonderful and healthy root vegetables: jicama, beets, and carrots.

INGREDIENTS | SERVES 2

2 cups peeled and grated jicama

1½ cups peeled and grated fresh beets

1½ cups peeled grated fresh carrots

Juice of 3 large lemons

3 tablespoons extra-virgin olive oil

1 teaspoon salt

1. In a medium salad bowl, combine the jicama, beets, and carrots.

2. In a small bowl, make the dressing by combining the lemon juice, olive oil, and salt. Whisk to combine the ingredients.

3. Pour the dressing on the salad. Toss to combine and serve.

Jicama

Jicama is a starchy root vegetable. You may find it in the produce section of your supermarket, or it can be easily found at Hispanic supermarkets.

Mint and Watermelon Salad

This is a refreshing salad that everyone will love. Simple and delicious, enjoy it sitting by the pool on a hot and sunny day.

INGREDIENTS | SERVES 4

5 cups cubed fresh watermelon

1½ cups chopped fresh mint

2 tablespoons minced fresh gingerroot

Juice of ½ medium lemon

1. In a large bowl, combine the watermelon, mint, ginger, and lemon juice. Mix to combine all ingredients.

2. Let the ingredients marry for 5 minutes in the fridge.

3. Serve cold.

Fun Variation

When available, combine yellow and red watermelons. The taste doesn't change, but your guests will be impressed with the color combination.

Ginger Turmeric Potato Salad

*This recipe combines all the flavors that you love from traditional potato salad,
with all the added health benefits of ginger and turmeric.*

INGREDIENTS | SERVES 4

3 cups Resistant Starch Potatoes (see
  recipe in Chapter 11), cut into cubes

2 medium stalks celery, diced

2 tablespoons chopped fresh dill

½ cup homemade mayonnaise

1 teaspoon ground ginger

1 teaspoon ground turmeric

1 teaspoon salt, or more to taste

1 teaspoon freshly ground black pepper

1. In a large salad bowl, combine the potatoes, celery, and dill.

2. Add the mayonnaise and stir to combine.

3. Add the ginger, turmeric, salt, and pepper. Stir again to combine all ingredients.

4. Taste the salad to see if it needs more salt. Serve.

Red Potatoes

This recipe works with any type of potatoes. However, it is recommended that you try using red potatoes with the skin on. It adds great color and the perfect combination of starch and buttery softness.

Spiced Egg Salad

Here is the classic egg salad with hints of turmeric, cayenne pepper, and smoked paprika.

INGREDIENTS | SERVES 4

8 large hard-boiled eggs

¾ cup homemade mayonnaise

¼ teaspoon cayenne pepper

¼ teaspoon ground ginger

1 teaspoon ground turmeric

1 teaspoon smoked paprika

1 teaspoon freshly ground black pepper

1 teaspoon salt, or more to taste

1. In a large salad bowl, mash the eggs using an egg masher.

2. Add the mayonnaise and stir to combine.

3. Add the cayenne pepper, ginger, turmeric, paprika, pepper, and salt. Stir again to combine all ingredients.

4. Serve.

Homemade Mayonnaise

Make sure to use homemade mayonnaise. Store-bought mayonnaise contains vinegar, which can produce excess mucus in the gut and contribute to inflammation. Homemade mayonnaise uses fresh lemon juice.

Ensalada de Jicama (Jicama Salad)

Refreshing, crispy, and spicy. Enjoy this salad with your favorite fish or grilled chicken recipe.

INGREDIENTS | SERVES 2

1 medium cucumber, peeled and cut into quarters

1 jalapeño pepper

¼ cup extra-virgin olive oil

¾ tightly packed cup fresh cilantro

2 tablespoons fresh lemon juice

½ teaspoon salt, or more to taste

½ teaspoon freshly ground black pepper

1 medium ripe avocado

2 medium jicamas peeled and julienned

Heat Level

This recipe is designed to be hot. If you prefer more of a mild to no heat, remove the seeds and veins from the jalapeño pepper.

1. In a blender, combine the cucumber, jalapeño, olive oil, cilantro, lemon juice, salt, and pepper.

2. Blend until the entire mixture has turned into liquid. If needed, add a little water to start blending. Taste the dressing for salt and add more if needed.

3. Cut the avocado into cubes and set aside.

4. Place the julienned jicama in a medium bowl.

5. Pour the dressing on the jicama and toss to make sure every slice of jicama is coated with the dressing.

6. Serve the salad in bowls and top each with half of the avocado. Sprinkle a pinch of salt on the avocado if desired.

Creamy Salmon Salad

This is a more sophisticated version of the classic tuna salad. Your family will love this recipe.

INGREDIENTS | SERVES 2

1 pound wild salmon fillet

Salt and freshly ground black pepper to taste

2 medium stalks celery, diced

¾ cup homemade mayonnaise

2 tablespoons chopped fresh dill

Juice of 1 medium lemon

Cooking Your Own Salmon

This recipe is best when you cook your own salmon for it. It makes a big difference in taste and quality. However, if you're on the go and need to make a faster meal, feel free to use canned salmon.

1. Preheat the oven to 375°F.

2. Place the salmon in a baking pan and season with salt and pepper. Bake for 30 minutes. Remove the salmon from the oven and allow it to cool for 10 minutes.

3. Shred the salmon off the skin, and place the shreds in a medium bowl.

4. Add the celery and mayonnaise and stir to combine.

5. Add the fresh dill, lemon juice, and salt and pepper to taste. Stir to combine. Serve immediately.

Yellow Mayonnaise Beet Slaw

This recipe uses the Turmeric Mayonnaise recipe found in this book (Chapter 13).
The turmeric adds a wonderful color and many health benefits.

INGREDIENTS | SERVES 4

5 large beets, peeled and grated

¾ cup homemade Turmeric Mayonnaise
(see recipe in Chapter 13)

¼ teaspoon ground ginger

1 teaspoon smoked paprika

1 teaspoon salt, or more to taste

1 teaspoon freshly ground black pepper

1. In a large salad bowl, combine the grated beets and turmeric mayonnaise. Using a wooden spoon, mix the salad.

2. Add the ginger, smoked paprika, salt, and pepper. Stir again to combine all the ingredients.

3. Taste the salad, and adjust seasonings to your liking. Serve.

Variation
Feel free to add other grated root vegetables such as parsnips or carrots to this recipe. You may also combine red and yellow beets for a festive presentation.

Mango and Jicama Salad

This salad is a sweet and crunchy mouth-watering combination
that will be the best complement to your grilled dishes.

INGREDIENTS | SERVES 2

3 tablespoons extra-virgin olive oil

Juice of 2 medium lemons

Salt and freshly ground black pepper to
taste

2 cups peeled and cubed jicama

2 cups cubed ripe mango

1 small purple onion, diced

¼ cup chopped fresh cilantro

1. In a small bowl, combine the oil, lemon juice, salt, and pepper.

2. In a large bowl, combine the jicama, mango, onion, and cilantro.

3. Add the dressing and toss the salad with a wooden spoon.

4. Taste the salad for salt and pepper. Serve immediately.

Full Vegetarian Meal
If you wish to make this meal a full vegetarian meal, add 2 cubed avocados. The avocado will add more texture and protein.

Roasted Beet Salad

Enjoy the sweetness and softness of roasted beets
in this magnificent salad with lemon-orange vinaigrette.

INGREDIENTS | SERVES 2

5 medium red beets, ends removed

¼ cup extra-virgin olive oil, plus extra
  for drizzling on the beets

Juice of 2 medium lemons

Juice of 2 medium oranges

Zest of ½ orange

Zest of 1 lemon

1 teaspoon salt

1 teaspoon freshly ground black pepper

1½ cups mixed greens

Yellow Beets

Add more color to this salad by replacing
half the red beets with yellow beets.

1. Preheat the oven to 375°F.

2. Place the beets on a piece of foil big enough to create
   a pouch.

3. Drizzle the olive oil on the beets and close the aluminum foil, creating a perfectly sealed pouch. Bake for
   45 minutes.

4. Remove the beets from the oven. Peel the beets and
   cut them into quarters.

5. Make the dressing by whisking together the citrus
   juices, zest, ¼ cup olive oil, salt, and pepper in a
   medium bowl.

6. Add the beets to the bowl with the dressing and stir.

7. Add the greens to the bowl and toss. Serve
   immediately.

Berry-Nutritious Antioxidant Salad

Some studies show that 1 cup of berries per day provides the necessary disease-fighting antioxidants that you need for 1 day.

INGREDIENTS | SERVES 2

1 cup cubed mango
1 cup blueberries
1 cup raspberries
1 cup sliced strawberries
Juice of ½ medium orange
Juice of 1 medium lemon
Fresh mint for garnish

1. In a large bowl, combine the mango, blueberries, raspberries, and strawberries.

2. Add the orange and lemon juice. Toss gently to combine.

3. Garnish with fresh mint. Serve immediately.

Add a Boost

When in season, add the seeds of one pomegranate to your salad. This will boost the antioxidant properties of your salad.

Spiced Apples and Bananas Dessert Salad

Enjoy this recipe for breakfast or for a healthy dessert option.

INGREDIENTS | SERVES 2

2 tablespoons fresh lemon juice
1 teaspoon raw honey
1 tablespoon ground cinnamon
1 teaspoon fresh-grated nutmeg
1 teaspoon pure vanilla extract
2 medium Gala apples, cored and diced
2 medium bananas, sliced (on the green side)
Fresh mint for garnish

1. In a small bowl, mix the lemon juice, honey, cinnamon, nutmeg, and vanilla extract to make a dressing.

2. In a medium bowl, combine the apples and bananas.

3. Add the dressing, and toss. Garnish with fresh mint and serve.

Asparagus Salad

The asparagus in this recipe is cut using a potato peeler,
but if you prefer you could also julienne the asparagus.

INGREDIENTS | SERVES 2

1 pound fresh asparagus, shaved with potato peeler

1 tablespoon chopped fresh Italian parsley

¼ cup extra-virgin olive oil

4 tablespoons fresh lemon juice

1 teaspoon lemon zest

Salt and freshly ground black pepper to taste

1. Place the shaved asparagus and parsley in a medium salad bowl.

2. In a small bowl, make the dressing by mixing the olive oil, lemon juice, lemon zest, salt, and pepper.

3. Add the dressing to the asparagus and toss. Taste for salt and pepper and add more if needed. Serve.

Classic Coleslaw

This is a classic, crunchy, creamy, and sweet dish. You can't go wrong with this coleslaw.

INGREDIENTS | SERVES 4

½ large head white cabbage, finely shredded

½ large head purple cabbage, finely shredded

2 large peeled carrots

1 cup homemade mayonnaise

1 tablespoon raw honey

Pinch of salt

1. Place the shredded cabbage and carrots in a large bowl.

2. Add the mayonnaise and honey. Stir with a spoon.

3. Add salt to taste.

Mayo-Free Variation

If you'd like a mayonnaise-free version of this coleslaw, combine ¼ cup lemon juice with ¼ cup olive oil, 1 tablespoon raw honey, and salt and pepper to taste. Whisk and add to the slaw instead of mayonnaise.

Endive and Heart of Palm Salad

The bitterness of the endives is well balanced with the tartness and freshness of the hearts of palm.

INGREDIENTS | SERVES 2

1 (16-ounce) can or jar of hearts of palm, sliced

4 large heads endive, bottoms removed and leaves separated

2 tablespoons extra-virgin olive oil

Juice of ½ medium lemon

Salt and freshly ground black pepper to taste

1. In a medium bowl, combine the hearts of palm and endive and toss to combine.

2. Separate the salad onto 2 serving plates.

3. Drizzle the olive oil and the juice of half lemon onto each plate.

4. Add salt and pepper to taste.

Add Avocado

This recipe taste great with avocado. Add 1 avocado cut into cubes to this salad for protein and a smooth texture.

Blood Orange and Arugula Salad

They say you eat with your eyes first. This salad will sure make your mouth waters just by looking at it.

INGREDIENTS | SERVES 2

Juice of 1 orange

Juice of 1 lemon

¼ cup extra-virgin olive oil

Salt and freshly ground black pepper to taste

2 cups fresh arugula

2 blood oranges, peeled and cut into long slices

Green onions, sliced for garnish

1. Combine the orange juice, lemon juice, oil, salt, and pepper in a small bowl. Whisk well to combine, or put in a blender.

2. In a large bowl, combine the arugula and sliced oranges. Pour the dressing onto the salad and toss. Garnish with green onions and serve.

CHAPTER 16

Vegetables

Turmeric and Dill Carrots
236

Roasted Root Vegetables
Medley
237

Sautéed Green Beans
with Fresh Garlic
238

Silky Parsnip Mash
239

Breakfast Zucchini
240

Spicy Asparagus
240

Parsnip and Celery Root Mash
241

Curly Carrot Strings
242

Shaved Zucchini and Carrots
243

Roasted Turmeric
Brussels Sprouts
244

Squash Blossom Stir-Fry
245

Pan-Fried Onions with
Fresh Thyme
246

Napa Cabbage Stir-Fry
247

Lemon and Pepper
Spaghetti Squash
248

Sautéed Mushrooms with Garlic
249

Sautéed Mushrooms
and Spinach
250

Turmeric and Dill Carrots

These carrots are a great side dish to any roasted chicken or grilled steak.

INGREDIENTS | SERVES 4

12 medium carrots peeled, sliced into
  ¼" pieces
2 tablespoons extra-virgin olive oil
1 tablespoon ground turmeric
1 teaspoon salt
1 teaspoon freshly ground black pepper
½ cup chopped fresh dill

Beta-Carotene

Carrots are a great source of beta-carotene, which is well known for its antioxidant properties. Some studies have found that eating foods rich in beta-carotene may have positive effects in reducing cardiovascular disease.

1. Preheat the oven to 375°F.

2. Put the carrots in a large baking pan. Add the olive oil, and mix well to combine.

3. Add the turmeric, salt, and pepper and combine to make sure every piece is coated with the spices.

4. Sprinkle on the fresh dill, and mix well to combine.

5. Place the baking pan in the oven, and cook for 30 minutes, or until the carrots are soft. Remove from the oven and serve warm.

Roasted Root Vegetables Medley

This is a delicious and fun way to eat root vegetables.
They are sweet, savory, crunchy, and perfect for any occasion.

INGREDIENTS | SERVES 4

8 young carrots with the green tops intact

8 medium parsnips, peeled and cut into long wedges

4 medium beets, peeled and quartered

2 tablespoons extra-virgin olive oil

2 sprigs fresh rosemary, leaves coarsely chopped

1 teaspoon salt

1 teaspoon freshly ground black pepper

Add More Color

If available, add purple carrots to this medley. If you're lucky you might also find white carrots. This will add more character to your dish and your family will love them!

1. Preheat the oven to 375°F.

2. Put the carrots, parsnips, and beets in a large baking pan.

3. Add the olive oil, and mix well to combine.

4. Add the chopped rosemary. Season with salt and pepper, and mix well.

5. Place the baking pan in the oven, and cook for 30 minutes, or until the vegetables are tender. Remove from the oven and serve warm.

Sautéed Green Beans with Fresh Garlic

Green beans are crunchy and delicious, great for any occasion, and good for your body.

INGREDIENTS | SERVES 4

2 tablespoons extra-virgin olive oil

1½ pounds fresh green beans, ends removed

2 cloves garlic, minced

1½ teaspoons salt

1 teaspoon freshly ground black pepper

1 medium lemon

Variation

Add more texture and flavor to this recipe by adding 1 diced medium shallot. This will add not only more texture but also more sweetness to this recipe.

1. Heat the oil in a large pan over medium heat.

2. Add the green beans and stir frequently for 3 minutes.

3. Add the fresh garlic and stir. Cook for another 3 minutes.

4. Season with salt and pepper, and mix well. Cook for another 2 minutes. The green beans should be crunchy; cook longer if you desire a softer texture.

5. Squeeze fresh lemon juice on the beans right before serving.

Silky Parsnip Mash

*This is a great way to enjoy the texture of mashed potatoes
without having all the carbohydrates of potatoes.*

INGREDIENTS | SERVES 2

1 pound parsnips, peeled and sliced

3 cloves garlic, mashed

1 bay leaf

½ cup water

1 cup light coconut milk, divided

Salt and freshly ground black pepper to
taste

2 tablespoons olive oil

2 tablespoons coconut oil

1 tablespoon ground turmeric

Make It Richer

Want to make this recipe richer and creamier? Replace ½ cup light coconut milk with
full-fat coconut milk. This will make your
parsnip mash creamier.

1. Place the parsnips, garlic, and bay leaf in a medium saucepan.

2. Add the water, ½ cup coconut milk, and salt and pepper to taste. Bring to a boil over medium-high heat.

3. As soon as the mixture begins to boil, reduce the heat to low and simmer for 15 minutes, or until the parsnips are tender.

4. Remove the bay leaf and strain the water. Transfer to a food processor.

5. Add the remaining coconut milk, olive oil, coconut oil, and turmeric to the food processor.

6. Blend until creamy and smooth. Add more salt and pepper if needed.

Breakfast Zucchini

Want to cut down on calories for breakfast? Use this recipe to replace breakfast potatoes.

INGREDIENTS | SERVES 2

2 tablespoons olive oil

3 large zucchini, diced

¼ cup chopped fresh dill

Salt and freshly ground black pepper to taste

1 tablespoon dried basil

1. Heat the oil in a large pan over medium heat.

2. Add the zucchini and fresh dill. Cook for 3 minutes, stirring occasionally. Season with salt and pepper.

3. Sprinkle with dried basil and cook for another 2 minutes.

4. Serve warm.

Spicy Kick

If you like a spicy kick, add some cayenne pepper to the zucchini a minute before they are fully cooked.

Spicy Asparagus

This recipe tastes great with grilled or pan-seared whitefish or salmon. Squeeze on some fresh lemon juice before eating.

INGREDIENTS | SERVES 2

2 tablespoons extra-virgin olive oil

1 pound asparagus, cut into thirds

1 clove garlic, minced

2 teaspoons red pepper flakes, or to taste

Salt and freshly ground black pepper to taste

Juice of 1 medium lemon

1. Heat the oil in a large pan over medium heat.

2. Add the asparagus and garlic to the hot pan and cook for 3 minutes, stirring occasionally.

3. Add the red pepper flakes, and salt and pepper to taste. Cook for another 3–4 minutes.

4. Remove from heat. Place the asparagus on large platter. Squeeze fresh lemon juice over the top and serve immediately.

Parsnip and Celery Root Mash

Here is another great way to cut down on the carbohydrates. This recipe has the combination of celery root and parsnip, great for both texture and taste.

INGREDIENTS | SERVES 4

1 pound parsnips, peeled and sliced

1 pound celery root, peeled and sliced

1 clove garlic

2 cups gluten-free chicken stock

2 tablespoons extra-virgin olive oil

2 tablespoons coconut oil

¾ cup light coconut milk

Salt and freshly ground black pepper to taste

Benefits of Celery Root

Celery root, also known as celeriac, is rich in antioxidants, vitamin K, minerals, and phosphorus, and is low in calories.

1. Place the parsnips, celery root, and garlic in a medium saucepan. Add the chicken stock and bring to a boil over medium-high heat. Cook for 5 minutes.

2. Reduce the heat to low and simmer for 15 minutes, or until the parsnips are tender. Remove from heat.

3. Place the mixture in a food processor, and save the juice.

4. Add the olive oil, coconut oil, and coconut milk, and enough of the parsnip juice to blend.

5. Blend until you have a smooth and silky texture. Season with salt and pepper to taste.

Curly Carrot Strings

A fun, tasty, and elegant way of eating carrots. During the winter months you may find purple and white carrots. Combine the colors to achieve a beautiful and colorful recipe.

INGREDIENTS | SERVES 4

9 large carrots, peeled

3 tablespoons olive oil

1 teaspoon ground ginger

2 tablespoons ground turmeric

Pinch cayenne pepper

Salt and freshly ground black pepper to taste

1. In a medium salad bowl, shave the carrots into long, flat strings using a potato peeler.

2. Heat the oil in a large pan over medium heat. Add the carrots to the hot oil.

3. Season immediately with ginger, turmeric, cayenne, salt, and pepper. Stir to make sure every string is coated with seasoning. Cook for 5 minutes, until the carrots are translucent.

4. Serve warm.

Shaved Zucchini and Carrots

Serve this with your favorite chicken or fish recipe. If you desire more texture, feel free to add some shaved parsnips, beets, or any vegetable that can be eaten raw and shaved using a potato peeler.

INGREDIENTS | SERVES 2

4 medium carrots peeled

4 medium green zucchini

3 tablespoons extra-virgin olive oil

1 tablespoon fresh lemon juice

Salt and freshly ground black pepper to taste

1. In a medium salad bowl, shave the carrots into long, flat strings using a potato peeler.

2. Using the same potato peeler, shave the zucchini.

3. Add the oil and lemon juice. Toss to mix together all the ingredients.

4. Season with salt and pepper to taste. Serve cold.

Roasted Turmeric Brussels Sprouts

These Brussels sprouts are crunchy and salty. Serve these with steak or chicken.

INGREDIENTS | SERVES 4

2 pounds Brussels sprouts

¼ cup extra-virgin olive oil

2 teaspoons salt

2 teaspoons freshly ground black pepper

1 tablespoon ground turmeric

Add Herbs

Add 1 tablespoon dried Herbes de Provence to this recipe for more flavor. Or you may simply add dried oregano and basil.

1. Preheat the oven to 400°F. Cut off the ends of the Brussels sprouts. Remove any black skin.

2. In a large bowl, combine the Brussels sprouts with the olive oil, salt, pepper, and turmeric. Toss together.

3. Transfer to a large baking pan. Place in the oven and roast for 35–40 minutes until soft and Brussels sprouts are brown.

4. Sprinkle with more salt if needed.

Squash Blossom Stir-Fry

When available, squash blossoms are a fun and gourmet vegetable to serve.
They are mild in flavor and easy to cook.

INGREDIENTS | SERVES 2

2 tablespoons extra virgin olive oil
2 medium shallots, chopped
30 squash blossoms, rinsed and dried
1 teaspoon salt
1 teaspoon freshly ground black pepper
1 teaspoon turmeric
2 tablespoons gluten-free chicken stock

Serve on Rice

This recipe is delicious served on a bed of Resistant Starch Brown Rice (see recipe in Chapter 11). Top it off with some avocado for a little protein.

1. Heat the oil over medium heat in a large pan.

2. Add the shallots and cook for 2 minutes, until translucent.

3. Immediately add the squash blossoms, and stir. Season with salt, pepper, and turmeric. Stir frequently and cook for 2 more minutes.

4. Add the chicken stock and stir. Most of the chicken stock will evaporate.

5. Cook for 5 minutes.

Pan-Fried Onions with Fresh Thyme

These are the perfect onions to use as a topping for burgers, steaks, or chicken.

INGREDIENTS | SERVES 4

2 tablespoons extra virgin olive oil

2–3 large white onions, sliced

1 teaspoon salt

1 teaspoon freshly ground black pepper

2 springs thyme, chopped

Variation

Want to get a stronger, spicy onion flavor? Simply replace the white onions with purple onions. These onions have a spicy flavor.

1. Heat the oil over medium heat in a large pan.

2. Add the onions and season with salt and pepper. Stir occasionally until the onions start to get soft, about 5 minutes.

3. Add the thyme. Continue stirring for a couple of minutes. The natural juices and sugars from the onions will begin to come out. Cook until the onions are brown in color approximately 8–10 minutes.

Napa Cabbage Stir-Fry

Napa cabbage is the perfect combination of crunchy and soft—perfect for stir-fry dishes or salads.

INGREDIENTS | SERVES 2

2 tablespoons extra virgin olive oil
3 medium carrots peeled and sliced
3 medium stalks celery, sliced
1 (1") piece fresh gingerroot, chopped
4 cups sliced napa cabbage
½ teaspoon salt
½ teaspoon freshly ground black pepper
2 tablespoons Braggs Liquid Aminos

1. Heat the oil over medium heat in a large pan.

2. Add the carrots and celery and cook for 2 minutes, stirring frequently.

3. Add the ginger and napa cabbage. Season with salt and pepper. Stir frequently and cook for 2 more minutes.

4. Add the Braggs Liquid Aminos, stir, and cook for 1 or 2 minutes until the carrots are al dente. Serve.

Serve with Fish

This recipe is delicious served with baked or pan-fried whitefish and Resistant Starch Brown Rice (see recipe in Chapter 11).

Lemon and Pepper Spaghetti Squash

*Spaghetti squash is an excellent and healthy alternative to regular noodles.
It is lower in calories but still gives you the texture of noodles.*

INGREDIENTS | SERVES 4

1 medium spaghetti squash

4 medium stalks celery, sliced

Juice of 2 medium lemons

Zest of 1 medium lemon

Salt and freshly ground black pepper to taste

¼ cup extra-virgin olive oil

2 teaspoons red pepper flakes

Bell Pepper Variation

If you don't have issues with bell pepper, add ½ cup of diced red bell pepper and ½ cup of diced green bell peppers to this recipe.

1. In a large pot boil enough water to cover the squash. Cut the squash in half lengthwise and add to the pot. Cook for 30 minutes, until soft.

2. Remove from heat, drain the water, and let the squash cool. Use a fork to remove the meat.

3. In a medium bowl, combine the squash meat, celery, lemon juice, lemon zest, and olive oil. Season with salt and pepper to taste.

4. Add the pepper flakes. Serve.

Sautéed Mushrooms with Garlic

Mushrooms offer a woody and smoky taste. This recipe works great with any mushroom, so feel free to use cremini, shiitake, oyster mushrooms, etc.

INGREDIENTS | SERVES 4

3 tablespoons olive oil

2 cloves garlic, minced

2 pounds white mushrooms, cleaned

Zest of 1 medium lemon

2 teaspoons red pepper flakes

Salt and freshly ground black pepper to taste

1. Heat the oil over medium heat in a large pan.

2. Add the garlic and sauté for 1 minute.

3. Immediately add the mushrooms and lemon zest and cook for 3 minutes, stirring occasionally.

4. Add the red pepper flakes. Stir until the mushrooms are fully cooked, about 2–3 minutes.

5. Add salt and pepper.

6. Serve.

Sautéed Mushrooms and Spinach

Make this recipe whenever you want a fast and easy vegetable side dish. It cooks in less than 10 minutes.

INGREDIENTS | SERVES 2

2 tablespoons extra-virgin olive oil

4 cups sliced white mushrooms

1 clove garlic, finely chopped

Salt and freshly ground black pepper to taste

4 cups fresh spinach

Asian-Style Variation

For an Asian variation of this dish, omit the salt, add 2 tablespoons chopped ginger-root, and season with Braggs Liquid Aminos. The Braggs will give it a soy sauce flavor.

1. In a large skillet over medium heat, heat the oil.

2. Add the mushrooms and garlic to the skillet and season with salt and pepper. Cook for 4 minutes, stirring frequently.

3. Add the spinach. The spinach will reduce in size in about 2 minutes.

4. Season the spinach with salt and pepper. Cook for 1 minute more.

CHAPTER 17

Snacks

Banana and Cacao Pudding
252

Raw Jicama Fries
253

Classic Guacamole
253

Turmeric-Spiced Kale Chips
254

Mango Sorbet
255

Spiced Poached Pears
256

Steamed Sweet Plantains
257

Crustless Apple Pie
258

L.A. Streets Fruit Salad
259

Turmeric Deviled Eggs
260

Watermelon and Ginger
Ice Cubes
261

Dates Stuffed with Chocolate
Coconut Butter
261

Figs with Coconut Cream
262

Baked Sweet Potato Cubes
262

Banana and Dates Shake
263

Banana and Cacao Pudding

If you are craving chocolate this healthy and creamy recipe will hit the spot!

INGREDIENTS | SERVES 2

3 large bananas

1 tablespoon coconut oil

2 tablespoons unsweetened cacao powder

Pinch of salt

1. In a medium bowl, mash the bananas with a potato masher.

2. Add the coconut oil and mash again to combine.

3. Add the cacao powder and mix well to combine all the ingredients.

4. Add a pinch of salt and mix.

5. Enjoy as is, or use it a dip for apple wedges.

Raw Jicama Fries

This crunchy and salty snack that you'll enjoy at any time of the day is simple to make and easy to pack in sandwich bags.

INGREDIENTS | SERVES 2

1 large jicama, peeled
1 medium lemon
Salt to taste

Add Some Heat!

In Mexico and some parts of Central America, chili powder is sprinkled on jicama. Feel free to add a little cayenne pepper for a nice kick.

1. Cut the peeled jicama into wedges. Put the wedges into a medium bowl.

2. Squeeze the lemon juice on the jicama fries and toss. Add salt to taste.

3. Enjoy cold.

Classic Guacamole

This is a recipe for a creamy, crunchy, and spicy guacamole with a touch of lemon.

INGREDIENTS | SERVES 3

3 large avocados
1 tablespoon extra-virgin olive oil
½ teaspoon salt
¼ teaspoon pepper.
1 tablespoon fresh lemon juice
¼ cup finely chopped purple onion
¼ cup finely chopped fresh cilantro
1 jalapeño pepper, seeded and chopped

Variation

If you don't have jalapeños available, sprinkle a dash of cayenne pepper or powdered chipotle to add some heat.

1. In a medium bowl, mash the avocadoes with a fork or potato masher.

2. Add the olive oil, salt, pepper, lemon juice, onion, cilantro, and jalapeño. Mix well to combine.

3. Taste for salt. Eat immediately.

Turmeric-Spiced Kale Chips

*These chips are a healthy alternative to potato chips. The turmeric adds
anti-inflammatory properties to this healthy snack.*

INGREDIENTS | SERVES 4

1 large head kale, washed and dried
3 tablespoons extra-virgin olive oil
1 tablespoon ground turmeric
1 teaspoon sea salt

1. Preheat the oven to 300°F.

2. Remove the ribs from the kale. Cut the kale into your
   favorite size for chips, ½–¾".

3. In a medium bowl, mix the kale, oil, turmeric, and salt.

4. Place the kale on a baking sheet. Bake for 10 minutes.

5. Turn the kale chips and cook for another 10 minutes or
   until the chips are crunchy.

Mango Sorbet

This is a healthy alternative to ice cream. You still get the satisfaction of eating something cold and creamy without all the calories and sugar of ice cream.

INGREDIENTS | SERVES 2

2 cups cubed frozen mango

2 medium bananas

¼ cup light coconut milk

Cold water if needed

Adding More Sweetness

If your mangoes are not sweet enough, and you desire a little more sweetness, add 1 tablespoon raw honey to your sorbet.

1. In a blender, combine the mango, bananas, and coconut milk. Blend until you have the consistency of sorbet.

2. If you're having difficulty blending, try adding 1 tablespoon of cold water. Add 1 tablespoon at a time until you get the blender going.

3. Serve immediately.

Spiced Poached Pears

To change the flavor of this dish to more of a sweeter, not-so-spicy combination, remove the cloves and peppercorns, and replace them with fresh vanilla beans.

INGREDIENTS | SERVES 4

2 sticks cinnamon
2 pieces fresh gingerroot cut in half
4 whole peppercorns
2 tablespoons raw honey
2 whole cloves
4 Anjou pears
Ground cinnamon for garnish

1. Boil enough water in a medium pan to cover all the pears.

2. Add the cinnamon sticks, ginger, peppercorns, honey, and cloves to the boiling water. Let the spices boil for 3 minutes.

3. Cover and reduce the heat to a simmer. Cook for 15 minutes.

4. While the spices are simmering, peel the pears, leaving the stem on. Core the pears from the bottom.

5. Place the pears in the simmering water. Increase the heat to medium. Cook the pears covered for 30 minutes.

6. Remove the pears from the heat and allow them to cool down for 10 minutes.

7. Serve the pears individually with some of the juices. Sprinkle with ground cinnamon.

Steamed Sweet Plantains

Similar to bananas in shape and taste, plantains are sweet and starchy. The extra starch makes them easy to cook.

INGREDIENTS | SERVES 2

2 large ripe plantains

2 tablespoons coconut oil

Ground cinnamon to taste

Buying Plantains

Plantains are available in most Hispanic supermarkets. Plantains with black spots are the best plantains to bake or fry. Yellow and soft plantains with not too many black spots are good for steaming.

1. Prepare a steamer.

2. Remove about ¼" off the ends of the plantains. Peel the plantains.

3. Place the plantains on the hot steamer. Cook for about 15–20 minutes or until the plantains are soft and cooked all the way to the center. Remove from heat.

4. Place the hot plantains on a serving dish. While still hot, drizzle 1 tablespoon coconut oil on top.

5. Sprinkle with ground cinnamon. Enjoy with hot tea or coffee.

Crustless Apple Pie

With this recipe, you'll enjoy the spices that you find in traditional apple pie, without the sugar and the wheat from the crust.

INGREDIENTS | SERVES 4

6 Granny Smith apples, peeled, cored, and thinly sliced

3 tablespoons coconut oil

3 tablespoons ground cinnamon

2 teaspoons freshly grated nutmeg

3 tablespoons vanilla extract

Apple Peel

This recipe calls for peeled apples. However, if you don't mind the peel, bake the apples with the skin on. Apple peel is loaded with fiber and nutrients that are beneficial to your health.

1. Preheat the oven to 375°F.

2. Place the sliced apples in a large baking pan.

3. Add the coconut oil, cinnamon, nutmeg, and vanilla extract. Mix all the apples by hand to make sure that every apple slice is coated with the spices.

4. Cover with aluminum foil. Bake for 1½ hours, until the apples are soft and falling apart.

5. Enjoy warm or cold.

L.A. Streets Fruit Salad

If you're ever in Los Angeles you'll find street vendors selling fresh fruit in plastic bags. This sweet, savory, and spicy combination will make your mouth water.

INGREDIENTS | SERVES 2

1 medium jicama, peeled and cut into long wedges

2 ripe mangoes, cored and cut into long wedges

2 cups cubed fresh watermelon

Meat of ½ coconut

1 large cucumber, cut in 8 wedges

Juice of 2 medium lemons

Salt to taste

Cayenne pepper to taste

Add Spices Before Serving

If you're not planning to eat this recipe immediately, place it in the fridge covered, with no spices or lemon juice added. Add the spices and lemon juice right before eating. This will prevent the fruit from getting soggy.

1. In a large bowl, combine the jicama, mangoes, watermelon, coconut meat, and cucumber.

2. Add the lemon juice and toss. Add salt and toss one more time.

3. Sprinkle with cayenne pepper to taste and serve immediately.

Turmeric Deviled Eggs

The classic deviled egg taste that you love with a boost of anti-inflammatory goodness from the turmeric.

INGREDIENTS | SERVES 3

6 jumbo eggs
1 tablespoon ground turmeric
¼ cup homemade mayonnaise
⅛ teaspoon salt
Freshly ground black pepper to taste
Smoked paprika for garnish

Variation

Want to add more taste and a little bit of crunch to this recipe? Add 1 tablespoon finely chopped onions or shallots.

1. Add the eggs to a medium saucepan. Add enough water to fully cover the eggs. Bring to a boil over medium heat and cook for 5 minutes.

2. Turn off the heat and leave covered for 10 more minutes. Remove the eggs from the hot water, and rinse with cold water. Let the eggs cool down for 5 minutes.

3. Once cool, peel the eggs and cut in half lengthwise.

4. Scoop out the egg yolks and place them in a medium bowl.

5. Put the egg whites on a serving platter.

6. Add the turmeric, mayonnaise, salt, and pepper to the eggs yolks. Mix until creamy.

7. Put a heaping spoonful of the yolk mixture into each egg white.

8. Sprinkle some smoked paprika for garnish.

Watermelon and Ginger Ice Cubes

Kids love this snack. The ginger provides anti-inflammatory properties as well as great digestive support. These are delicious any time of the day.

INGREDIENTS | SERVES 2

4 cups cubed sweet watermelon
3" piece of fresh gingerroot, peeled
¼ cup chopped fresh mint
Juice of 1 medium lemon
Pinch salt
1 tablespoon raw honey

1. In a blender, combine the watermelon, ginger, mint, lemon, salt, and honey. Blend until you have a smoothie texture.

2. Fill up 2 ice-cube trays with mixture. Freeze overnight.

3. Remove the cubes and eat cold.

Watermelon Sparking Water
Mix 4 watermelon cubes with 8 ounces of plain sparkling water for a refreshing and bubbly drink.

Dates Stuffed with Chocolate Coconut Butter

The natural sweetness of the dates combines with the delicious creamy texture of coconut butter to create a recipe you are sure to love.

INGREDIENTS | MAKES 6 DATES

6 Medjool dates
4 tablespoons coconut butter
1 tablespoon unsweetened cacao powder

1. Cut a slit on the side of each of the dates and remove the pits. Set pitted dates aside.

2. In a small bowl, mix the coconut butter with the cacao powder.

3. Using a small spoon, stuff the coconut butter mixture into each date. Serve immediately.

Coconut Butter
Coconut butter is made by combining the coconut meat with the coconut oil. It is perfect for desserts.

Figs with Coconut Cream

This is a great snack to enjoy at any time of the day. Healthy, simple, and tasty.

INGREDIENTS | SERVES 2

8 large fresh, ripe figs
¾ cup light coconut milk

1. Cut the figs into quarters and place in a medium bowl.

2. Add the coconut milk. Stir the dates to make sure that each piece is covered in milk.

3. Let the figs rest for 3 minutes before serving. This process will allow the juices to mix in with the milk.

Variation

Figs are naturally sweet, but sometimes you may encounter some figs that are not sweet enough. Add 1 tablespoon raw honey to add some sweetness to this snack if desired.

Baked Sweet Potato Cubes

Enjoy these cubes hot or cold.

INGREDIENTS | SERVES 4

3 large sweet potatoes, peeled and cubed
2 tablespoons extra-virgin olive oil
2 tablespoons coconut oil, melted
2 tablespoons ground cinnamon

1. Preheat the oven to 375°F.

2. Place the cubed sweet potatoes in a large baking pan. Drizzle the olive oil and coconut oil on the sweet potatoes. Mix well to make sure that every piece is coated with oil.

3. Add the cinnamon and mix well.

4. Bake for 40–45 minutes, until the sweet potatoes are soft.

Make It a Purée

This recipe works great as a purée. When the sweet potatoes are cooked, mash them and add a little more coconut oil and cinnamon.

Banana and Dates Shake

With this recipe bananas will never go to waste. The perfect bananas for this recipe are those that are on the green side, so as to avoid them being too ripened.

INGREDIENTS | SERVES 2

3 medium bananas, peeled and frozen for at least 4 hours or overnight

3 Medjool dates, pitted

1 cup light coconut milk

2 teaspoons ground cinnamon

1 cup coconut water, divided

1. Place the frozen bananas in a large blender. Add the dates, coconut milk, cinnamon, and ½ cup coconut water.

2. Blend on high for 1 minute, until the dates and bananas are fully blended. Add more coconut water if the consistency is too thick.

CHAPTER 18

Beverages

Golden Triangle Milk
266

Spiked Holy Basil Tea
267

Liquid Salsa
267

Red Head
268

Cherry Fire Extinguisher
269

Ginger Cooler
269

Golden Triangle Milk

This trio of anti-inflammatory herbs empowers this refreshing drink with powerful healing properties that are bound to help quench the fires of autoimmunity.

INGREDIENTS | SERVES 1

⅓ cup turmeric
2 teaspoons ground cinnamon
2 teaspoons ground ginger
1 cup water
1 cup light coconut milk

Look Out for Stains

Turmeric can stain the clothing, so wear an apron to protect your clothes.

1. Add the turmeric, cinnamon, ginger, and water to a small saucepan. Heat over medium heat for 7–10 minutes to create a paste. Add more water if necessary to reach a paste consistency.

2. Let cool. Store in a glass container in the refrigerator for up to 10 days. (The longer it is stored, the more bitter it may become.)

3. Add the coconut milk to a small saucepan.

4. Add 1 teaspoon turmeric paste to the pan and heat on medium heat for 3–5 minutes. Remove and drink as a tea or pour over ice for a cool treat.

Spiked Holy Basil Tea

Holy basil is regarded as the queen of herbs in India.
Feel free to use other species of basil in this recipe too.

INGREDIENTS | SERVES 2

2 cups water
2 tablespoons chopped holy basil
½ teaspoon grated fresh gingerroot

1. Bring the water to a boil.

2. Add the basil and ginger to a teapot and pour the hot water over them.

3. Cover and let steep for 10 minutes. Remove the cover and strain out the basil and ginger. Enjoy!

Guru in a Cup

In Ayurvedic medicine, holy basil helps to achieve deep meditative states, heightens awareness, imparts compassion, and increases mental clarity. It's enough to make a guru out of anyone. Note: Make sure that your followers drink it too, as it bestows devotion.

Liquid Salsa

This smoothie combines the anti-inflammatory properties of pineapple, cilantro, turmeric, and ginger with the cooling effect of avocados.

INGREDIENTS | SERVES 2

1 medium avocado
1 cup chopped pineapple
¼ cup chopped fresh cilantro
½ tablespoon virgin coconut oil
½ teaspoon turmeric
½ teaspoon minced ginger
1 cup light coconut milk

Place all the ingredients in a blender and blend for 45 seconds. Add ice for coolness and to thin the smoothie a bit.

Avocado Myth

The Mayan and Inca Indians assigned magical and mystical properties to avocados that included its ability to bestow sexual mastery upon whomever consumed it.

Red Head

Vivacious red beets make this drink dynamite, and the betaine substance found in beets provides plenty of strong anti-inflammatory properties.

INGREDIENTS | SERVES 2

¾ cup steamed red beets

2 cups raspberries

1 cup coconut milk

1 teaspoon turmeric

1 teaspoon ground ginger

1 tablespoon virgin coconut oil

¼ cup water

Add all the ingredients to a blender and blend until the desired consistency is reached.

Sweeter Beets

Oven-roasting beets will increase their sweetness. Clean and cut beets into ½"-thick slices, place on an aluminum-covered baking sheet, and lightly coat with coconut oil. Cover with aluminum foil and bake at 425°F for 60–90 minutes, until tender to a fork. Remove and allow to cool. After cooling, remove skins.

Cherry Fire Extinguisher

Tart cherries have been shown to contain compounds that deliver a powerful anti-inflammatory punch. Researchers at Oregon Health & Science University state that tart cherries "have the highest anti-inflammatory content of any food, including blueberries, pomegranates, and other fruits."

INGREDIENTS | SERVES 2

1 cup pitted tart cherries

1 cup light coconut milk

½ cup blueberries

½ teaspoon turmeric

½ teaspoon ground ginger

2 tablespoons virgin coconut oil

Add all the ingredients to a blender, adding the coconut oil last. Blend until smooth. Pour into a glass and enjoy with a blueberry or cherry garnish.

Ginger Cooler

Ginger is one of the stronger anti-inflammatory herbs that can easily be added to many foods and drinks. Ginger will spice up the flavor of dishes while reducing tummy troubles and cooling the inflammation associated with many diseases.

INGREDIENTS | SERVES 2

2" piece fresh gingerroot

2 cups water

2 cups ice

Mint leaves

1. Finely chop or grate the gingerroot and add to a medium bowl.

2. Boil the water and pour over the ginger. Cover and allow to steep for 20 minutes.

3. Place the ice into 2 cups and pour the ginger mixture over the ice.

4. Garnish with mint.

CHAPTER 19

Juicing

The Turmeric Original
272

Sweet and Spicy
272

Kidney Cleanser
273

Sweet Pepper
273

Green Beauty
274

Detox Special
274

Beet and Fennel Blood
Strengthener
275

Infection Fighter
275

Cheerful Broccoli
276

Super Immune System
276

Fine and Dandy-lion
277

Digestive Aid
277

Spicy Ginger Charmer
278

Cherry Lemonade
279

Inflammation Be Gone
279

Spicy Peppermint Shot
280

The Turmeric Original

This tasty drink contains the centuries-old wonder herb turmeric, known for its inflammation-fighting properties and colorful presence. Make turmeric a part of your daily diet for best results.

INGREDIENTS | SERVES 1

1" turmeric root
⅓ lemon with rind
4 medium carrots
1 green apple, cored

Add all the ingredients to a juicer in the order listed. Drink right away.

Sweet and Spicy

Parsley is the long-time nemesis of many diseases, including autoimmune ones. Its antioxidant benefits are aided by the addition of ginger to this wonderfully simple, yet potent anti-inflammatory mixture.

INGREDIENTS | SERVES 1

½ handful fresh Italian parsley
1" piece fresh gingerroot
1½ pears, cored
1 green apple, cored

Add all the ingredients to a juicer in the order listed. Drink right away.

Individual Tastes

Ginger is a powerful anti-inflammatory herb that can be increased in this drink according to each person's taste and tolerance. Play around with the amount to see if more is better, although that's not always the case.

Kidney Cleanser

Kale has antioxidant and anticancer properties that make it a wonderful addition to any autoimmune diet protocol.

INGREDIENTS | SERVES 1

3 kale leaves

1 cup cranberries

1½ cups grapes

2" pineapple round

Add all the ingredients to a juicer in the order listed. Drink right away.

Oily Benefits

Coconut oil can make a good addition to any juice recipe. It can slow down metabolism of fruit sugars, while also providing some nice antimicrobial properties that can help support better gut health. Experiment with ⅛ cup in your juice recipes.

Sweet Pepper

The colorful bell pepper contains carotenoids that help boost, maintain, and modulate immune system function. The lutein and zeaxanthin in bell peppers can help reduce inflammation.

INGREDIENTS | SERVES 1

3 medium carrots

½ medium green bell pepper, seeded

¾ medium cucumber

½ medium green apple, cored

Add all the ingredients to a juicer in the order listed. Drink right away.

Risk versus Benefit

Bell peppers are a member of the nightshade family, which many people recommend avoiding on an autoimmune diet. On the other hand, they are high in vitamins A and C and antioxidants that fight inflammation.

Green Beauty

If there's one color that's always associated with health, it's the color green. This concoction is loaded with vitamins and minerals that support immunity. The addition of cucumbers helps support hair, nails, and especially the skin. There's no need to skimp on beauty while getting healthier!

INGREDIENTS | SERVES 1

½ handful fresh Italian parsley

2 large kale leaves

½–1 medium pear

3 medium celery stalks

1 medium cucumber

Add all the ingredients to a juicer in the order listed. Drink right away.

Green Smoothie

Convert this wonderful green drink into a smoothie by adding ½ an avocado and a cup of ice with the juice and blending them together in a blender. It makes for a creamy, refreshing drink any time of the year.

Detox Special

This is a tasty way to reduce the body's toxic load of chemicals. The high levels of chlorophyll in this recipe will aid the body in eliminating toxins while restoring life to the cells.

INGREDIENTS | SERVES 1

½ handful fresh Italian parsley

1" piece gingerroot

4 medium carrots

1 medium green apple

Add all the ingredients to a juicer in the order listed. Drink right away.

Beet and Fennel Blood Strengthener

The beets in this drink are a strong tonic for the blood and assist in detoxification. Aided by the blood-strengthening effects of fennel, this mixture becomes a potent remedy for many ills.

INGREDIENTS | SERVES 1

1 medium beet with greens
1 clove garlic
½ fennel bulb with green stalks
1½ medium green apples

Add all the ingredients to a juicer in the order listed. Drink right away.

Infection Fighter

With the anxiety and stress reducing benefits of celery combined with the antimicrobial properties of garlic, this concoction is an excellent mind-body aid for whole health.

INGREDIENTS | SERVES 1

½ handful fresh Italian parsley
1 clove garlic
4 medium carrots
5 medium stalks celery

Add all the ingredients to a juicer in the order listed. Drink right away.

Take It Up a Notch

For additional immune system benefits, try adding some turmeric and ginger to help cool the fires of inflammation, while promoting better digestion.

Cheerful Broccoli

A good disposition can help chase away the blues and stress. Broccoli contains powerful substances, sulforaphane and indole, that fight cancers. An additional benefit of indole is its ability to manage estrogen levels.

INGREDIENTS | SERVES 1

3 large kale leaves

½ small head broccoli

4 medium carrots

1 medium green apple, cored

Add all the ingredients to a juicer in the order listed. Drink right away.

Super Immune System

The sulfur compounds contained in onions help power detoxification pathways in the body, while onion's quercetin levels exert their anti-inflammatory and antihistamine effects. The chromium in onions also helps balance blood sugar issues.

INGREDIENTS | SERVES 1

½ handful fresh Italian parsley

1 beet with greens

¼ red onion

3 medium carrots

2 medium stalks celery

1 medium green apple, cored

Add all the ingredients to a juicer in the order listed. Drink right away.

Fine and Dandy-lion

The addition of chia seeds to this recipe helps slow the breakdown of carbohydrates and absorption of sugar to decrease inflammation.

INGREDIENTS | SERVES 1

¼ bunch dandelion greens

1½ cups grapes

2 kiwifruit

½ green apple, cored

½ tablespoon chia seeds

Add all the ingredients to a juicer in the order listed. Drink right away.

Alternate Choice

Flaxseeds can also be used in place of chia seeds, as both seeds will form a gel that helps promote regular bowel movements.

Digestive Aid

Almost every autoimmune condition is going to have some degree of digestive difficulty associated with it one way or another. With the addition of the Peruvian superfood maca, this juice becomes a great way to assist the body in regaining balance and better function.

INGREDIENTS | SERVES 1

8 large strawberries

15 tart cherries, seeded

¾ cup coconut water

1 teaspoon maca

1 teaspoon ground cinnamon

Add all the ingredients to a juicer in the order listed. Drink right away.

Superfoods

Superfoods are foods that are packed with a concentrated assortment of vitamins, minerals, antioxidants, and polyphenols. Each of the ingredients in this recipe is a superfood, so drink to your health, often!

Spicy Ginger Charmer

When you need to protect against toxins in the environment, inflammation in the body, radiation toxicity, digestive upset, and imbalances caused by blood sugar swings, it's time to get serious about ginger. Its 2,000-year history of benefits make it a wonder herb in autoimmunity.

INGREDIENTS | SERVES 1

⅛ bunch fresh cilantro

2" piece ginger

⅓ lemon with rind

1 medium tomato

2 medium carrots

¼ teaspoon cayenne pepper

¾ cup coconut water

Add all the ingredients to a juicer in the order listed. Drink right away.

Fat Science

Turning this recipe into a smoothie can be a useful way to assist the body in binding heavy metals and chemicals that are released due to the beneficial effects of cilantro. Try adding some beneficial fats like coconut oil, coconut butter, or ½ an avocado and blending with the juice for a fantastic smoothie.

Cherry Lemonade

Cherries will help calm the mind and body, while also reducing inflammation and laying the foundation for a relaxing day of work or a good night's sleep.

INGREDIENTS | SERVES 1

½ lemon with rind

15 cherries, seeded

1 cup coconut water

1 tablespoon apple cider vinegar

Add all the ingredients to a juicer in the order listed. Drink right away.

Cherry Delight

Turn this drink into a wonderful smoothie by thickening it with coconut oil or coconut butter and a cup of ice.

Inflammation Be Gone

This small shot will help chase away inflammation and leave the body feeling refreshed and energized with the zing of ginger, the refreshing flavor of lemon, the cooling effect of turmeric, and the superb healing qualities of apple cider vinegar.

INGREDIENTS | SERVES 1

¼ lemon with rind

¼ teaspoon ground turmeric

1" piece gingerroot

2 tablespoons apple cider vinegar

Add all the ingredients to a juicer in the order listed. Drink right away.

Spicy Peppermint Shot

When you need just a little boost that packs a big punch, this shot is the way to go.

INGREDIENTS | SERVES 1

½ handful fresh Italian parsley
10 peppermint leaves
2" piece fresh gingerroot
¼ teaspoon ground turmeric
¼ teaspoon ground cinnamon
2 tablespoons apple cider vinegar

Add all the ingredients to a juicer in the order listed. Drink right away.

Let Me Count the Ways

The use of apple cider vinegar has been around for centuries. It has twenty, thirty, fifty, or more uses depending on the authority consulted, which makes it an indispensible tool for healing and maintaining health in the body.

APPENDIX A

Resources

General Information

American Autoimmune Related Diseases Association (AARDA)
www.aarda.org

Environmental Working Group (EWG)
www.ewg.org

Estrogenic Activity Database (EADB)
www.fda.gov/ScienceResearch/BioinformaticsTools/EstrogenicActivityDatabaseEADB/default.htm

Occupational Safety and Health Administration
www.osha.gov/dsg/hazcom/finalmsdsreport.html

Centers for Disease Control and Prevention
www.cdc.gov

Integrative Oncology Consultants
www.moshefrenkelmd.com

Spontaneous Remission: An Annotated Bibliography
http://noetic.org/library/publication-books/spontaneous-remission-annotated-bibliography/

The Radical Remission Project
www.radicalremission.com

Dr. David Berceli's Tension and Trauma Release Exercises
www.traumaprevention.com

Dr. Peter A. Levine's Somatic Experiencing
www.somaticexperiencing.com

Dr. Stephen Porges's The Polyvagal Theory
www.amazon.com/Polyvagal-Theory-Neurophysiological-Communication-Self-regulation/
dp/0393707008

Dr. McCombs's Candida Diet
www.candidaplan.com

American Gut Project
www.americangut.org

Blue Zones Study
www.bluezones.com

Helminth Worm Therapy
www.wormtherapy.com

Dr. Datis Kharrazian's Autoimmune Blog
www.drknews.com

Celiac Disease Foundation
http://celiac.org/live-gluten-free/glutenfreediet/sources-of-gluten

Gluten Intolerance Group
www.gluten.org

Pickl-It Anaerobic Fermentation Supplies
www.Pickl-It.com

Gluten-Free Dining Guides

GlutenFree Passport
http://glutenfreepassport.com/allergy-gluten-free-restaurants/fast-food-chains-allergy-charts

Gluten*free* Restaurant Guides
http://glutenfreeguidehq.com/chain-restaurants

Gluten-Free Restaurant Menus from GlutenFreeTravelSite.com
http://glutenfreetravelsite.com/restaurants

Gluten-Free Living
www.glutenfreeliving.com/gluten-free-foods/diet/basic-diet

Gluten Testing

EnteroLab
www.enterolab.com
(972) 686-6869

Cyrex Laboratories
www.cyrexlabs.com
United States
(877) 772-9739
(602) 759-1245
United Kingdom
+44 (0)333 9000 979
Ireland
+44 (0)333 9000 979

TrueHealthLabs.com
www.truehealthlabs.com
(888) 763-1223

Sample Meal Plans

Week 1:

Sunday
Breakfast: Crustless Spinach and Potato Quiche (Chapter 10)
Lunch: Refreshing Avocado Soup (Chapter 14)
Dinner: Spanish Lamb Steaks with Silky Parsnip Mash (Chapters 12 and 16)
Dessert: Banana and Cacao Pudding (Chapter 17)
Snack: Turmeric-Spiced Kale Chips (Chapter 17)

Monday
Breakfast: Sweet Start Breakfast Porridge (Chapter 10)
Lunch: Leftover Crustless Spinach and Potato Quiche
Dinner: The Perfect Salmon Burgers (Chapter 12)
Dessert: 1 cup mixed berries
Snack: Cherry Lemonade (Chapter 19)

Tuesday
Breakfast: Spicy Kale Scramble (Chapter 10)
Lunch: Chicken and Brown Rice Salad (Chapter 15)
Dinner: Beef with Butternut Squash Stew (Chapter 14)
Dessert: Figs with Coconut Cream (Chapter 17)
Snack: Pumpkin Spice Applesauce (Chapter 13)

Wednesday
Breakfast: Banana and Dates Shake (Chapter 17)
Lunch: Leftover Beef with Butternut Squash Stew
Dinner: Casablanca Chicken Skewers (Chapter 12)
Dessert: 1 cup pineapple sprinkled with 2 tablespoons toasted coconut flakes
Snack: Spicy Ginger Charmer (Chapter 19)

Thursday
Breakfast: Super Immune System (Chapter 19)
Lunch: Chicken Salad with Apples and Grapes (Chapter 15)
Dinner: Squash Blossom Stir-Fry and Resistant Starch Brown Rice Pasta (Chapters 16 and 11)
Dessert: 2 slices honeydew melon
Snack: Raw Jicama Fries (Chapter 17)

Friday

Breakfast: Protein Power Breakfast (Chapter 10)

Lunch: Leftover Squash Blossom Stir-Fry and Resistant Starch Brown Rice Pasta

Dinner: Cucumber Mint Soup (Chapter 14)

Dessert: Spiced Apples and Bananas Dessert Salad (Chapter 15)

Snack: Baked Sweet Potato Cubes (Chapter 17)

Saturday

Breakfast: Farmer's Egg Casserole (Chapter 10)

Lunch: Ojai Ginger Lemon Salmon (Chapter 11)

Dinner: Perfect and Tender Pot Roast (Chapter 12)

Dessert: Mango Sorbet (Chapter 17)

Snack: Classic Guacamole (Chapter 17) with cucumber slices

Week 2:

Sunday

Breakfast: Turkey Breakfast Sausages (Chapter 10) with 1 fried egg

Lunch: Whitefish Soup (Chapter 14)

Dinner: Hugo's Carne Asada–Style Flank Steak (Chapter 12), served over Resistant Starch Brown Rice (Chapter 11) with steamed vegetable of choice

Dessert: Crustless Apple Pie (Chapter 17)

Snack: Turmeric Deviled Eggs (Chapter 17)

Monday

Breakfast: Bite-Sized Smoked Salmon Frittatas (Chapter 10)

Lunch: Leftover Turkey Breakfast Sausages served over 1 cup mixed greens

Dinner: Moroccan-Inspired Sea Bass (Chapter 12)

Dessert: 1 cup raspberries

Snack: Leftover Turmeric Deviled Eggs

Tuesday

Breakfast: Green Beauty (Chapter 19)

Lunch: Leftover Bite-Sized Smoked Salmon Frittatas

Dinner: Chicken breasts marinated in Indian-Inspired Chicken Marinade (Chapter 13) with Resistant Starch Brown Rice (Chapter 11) and steamed vegetable of choice

Dessert: Leftover Crustless Apple Pie

Snack: Steamed Sweet Plantains

Wednesday

Breakfast: Berry-Nutritious Antioxidant Salad (Chapter 15)

Lunch: Mediterranean Turkey Burger (Chapter 11)

Dinner: Butternut Squash Soup (Chapter 14)

Dessert: L.A. Streets Fruit Salad (Chapter 17)

Snack: Sweet Pepper (Chapter 19)

Thursday

Breakfast: Brown Rice Frittata (Chapter 10)

Lunch: Leftover Mediterranean Turkey Burger

Dinner: Salmon fillet with Lemon and Pepper Spaghetti Squash (Chapter 16)

Dessert: Dates Stuffed with Chocolate Coconut Butter (Chapter 17)

Snack: Leftover L.A. Streets Fruit Salad

Friday

Breakfast: Scrambled eggs with The Perfect Breakfast Potatoes (Chapter 10)

Lunch: Leftover Butternut Squash Soup

Dinner: Sizzling Grilled Lamb Chops (Chapter 12)

Dessert: Leftover Dates Stuffed with Chocolate Coconut Butter

Snack: Detox Special (Chapter 19)

Saturday

Breakfast: Spiced Poached Pears (Chapter 17)

Lunch: Roasted Root Vegetables Medley (Chapter 16)

Dinner: Asparagus Salad (Chapter 15) with sliced chicken thighs

Dessert: Mint and Watermelon Salad (Chapter 15)

Snack: Banana and Dates Shake (Chapter 17)

Week 3:

Sunday
Breakfast: Fluffy Yellow Turmeric Scrambled Eggs (Chapter 10)
Lunch: *Tom Kha Gai* Soup (Thai Coconut Chicken Soup) (Chapter 14)
Dinner: Pan-Seared Salmon with Oregano (Chapter 12)
Dessert: Mango Sorbet (Chapter 17)
Snack: 1 cup cherry tomatoes

Monday
Breakfast: Fine and Dandy-lion (Chapter 19)
Lunch: *Tortilla Española* (Spanish Omelet) (Chapter 11)
Dinner: Indian-Spiced Chicken Tenders (Chapter 12)
Dessert: Banana and Cacao Pudding (Chapter 17)
Snack: Leftover Mango Sorbet

Tuesday
Breakfast: Leftover *Tortilla Española* (Spanish Omelet)
Lunch: Chicken and Cauliflower Stir-Fry (Chapter 11)
Dinner: Ginger Turmeric Potato Salad (Chapter 15) with salad
Dessert: Leftover Banana and Cacao Pudding
Snack: Watermelon and Ginger Ice Cubes (Chapter 17)

Wednesday
Breakfast: Resistant Starch Porridge (Chapter 10)
Lunch: Peruvian Ceviche (Chapter 11)
Dinner: Coconut Cream of Broccoli Soup (Chapter 14)
Dessert: 1 sliced banana drizzled with 2 teaspoons raw honey
Snack: Classic Guacamole (Chapter 17) with sliced carrot sticks

Thursday
Breakfast: Salvadoran *Huevos Picados con Ejotes* (Green Bean Scramble) (Chapter 10)
Lunch: Harvest Chicken Soup (Chapter 11)
Dinner: Lemon Pepper Whitefish (Chapter 12)
Dessert: Figs with Coconut Cream (Chapter 17)
Snack: Infection Fighter (Chapter 19)

Friday
Breakfast: Poached Eggs and Porridge (Chapter 10)
Lunch: Leftover Harvest Chicken Soup
Dinner: Grilled steak of choice with Mango and Jicama Salad (Chapter 15)
Dessert: 1 cup mixed berries
Snack: Sweet and Spicy (Chapter 19)

Saturday
Breakfast: Breakfast Zucchini (Chapter 16) with 1 hard-boiled egg
Lunch: Sunny California Beet Salad (Chapter 11)
Dinner: Seared Ahi Tuna Steaks (Chapter 12)
Dessert: 1 sliced apple sprinkled with cinnamon
Snack: Spicy Asparagus (Chapter 16)

Week 4:

Sunday
Breakfast: Sweet Start Breakfast Porridge (Chapter 10)
Lunch: Herbes de Provence–Crusted Bison Sirloin Tip (Chapter 11)
Dinner: Turmeric Rice and Chicken (Chapter 12)
Dessert: Mint and Watermelon Salad (Chapter 15)
Snack: Digestive Aid (Chapter 19)

Monday
Breakfast: Breakfast Fried Rice (Chapter 10)
Lunch: Beet and Peach Salad (Chapter 11)
Dinner: Grilled shrimp in Cilantro Lime Marinade (Chapter 13)
Dessert: Mango Sorbet (Chapter 17)
Snack: Leftover Mint and Watermelon Salad

Tuesday
Breakfast: Crustless Spinach and Potato Quiche (Chapter 10)
Lunch: Pollo Verde (Green Chicken) (Chapter 11)
Dinner: Russian Salmon Soup (Chapter 14)
Dessert: L.A. Streets Fruit Salad (Chapter 17)
Snack: Turmeric Deviled Eggs (Chapter 17)

Wednesday
Breakfast: Banana and Dates Shake (Chapter 17)
Lunch: Leftover Crustless Spinach and Potato Quiche
Dinner: Spanish Lamb Steaks (Chapter 12)
Dessert: Leftover L.A. Streets Fruit Salad
Snack: Turmeric-Spiced Kale Chips (Chapter 17)

Thursday
Breakfast: Resistant Starch Porridge (Chapter 10)
Lunch: *Ensalada de Jicama* (Jicama Salad) (Chapter 15) with leftover Spanish Lamb Steaks
Dinner: Vegetable and Egg Soup (Chapter 14)
Dessert: 1 cup sliced strawberries topped with ⅛ cup toasted almonds
Snack: Spicy Peppermint Shot (Chapter 19)

Friday
Breakfast: Farmer's Egg Casserole (Chapter 10)
Lunch: Beet Soup (Chapter 14)
Dinner: Herbes de Provence–Crusted Halibut (Chapter 12)
Dessert: Spiced Poached Pears (Chapter 17)
Snack: Sweet and Spicy (Chapter 19)

Saturday
Breakfast: The Tumeric Original (Chapter 19) with 1 cup sliced pineapple
Lunch: Leftover Farmer's Egg Casserole
Dinner: Casablanca Chicken Skewers (Chapter 12)
Dessert: Spiced Apples and Bananas Dessert Salad (Chapter 15)
Snack: Baked Sweet Potato Cubes (Chapter 17)

Index

Note: Page numbers in **bold** indicate recipe category lists.

Acid reflux, 61–62
Adaptive response. *See* Specific immunity
Addison's disease, 16, 67
Age, autoimmune diseases and, 21–22
Aging, immune system and, 40
Aioli, 199
Allergens, 127
Aloo Gobi (Cauliflower and Potatoes), 177
Alpha lipoic acid (ALA), 114
ALS (alpha lipoic acid), 114
American Gut Project, 101, 102–3, 283
Andrographis (*Andrographis paniculata*), 117–18
Anemias, 15, 16, 17, 18, 113, 114, 140
Antibiotics
  autoimmune diseases and, 41
  fungal infections and, 95. *See also* Candida (*Candida albicans*)
  good and bad of, 92–95
  gut health and, 58, 96–97
  historical perspective, 92–95
  LPS and, 95–97
  resistance to, 29, 94
  risk-to-benefit considerations, 29
Antibodies
  about, 38–39
  aging and, 40
  B cells and, 14, 36
  to body's own tissue, 35, 40
  definition of autoimmune disease and, 16
  frankincense (*Boswellia serrata*) and, 118
  gluten, 140
  mercury and, 50
  selenium deficiency and, 116
  testing for, 22, 64
  types and functions, 38
Apples
  about: benefits of, 130, 258; nutrients in peel, 258
  Beet and Fennel Blood Strengthener (juice), 275

Chicken Salad with Apples and Grapes, 224
Crustless Apple Pie, 258
Detox Special (juice), 274
Pumpkin Spice Applesauce, 201
Spiced Apples and Bananas Dessert Salad, 232
Sweet and Spicy (juice), 272
Argentinean Steak Chimichurri, 200
Artichokes, benefits of, 130
Asian Marinade, 203
Asparagus
  Asparagus Salad, 233
  Spicy Asparagus, 240
Asthma, 34, 57, 95, 98, 103, 120, 124, 135
Autoimmune attacks
  direct, 66–67
  "enemy" within and, 27
  immune system toolbox and, 31–39
  medication and, 41
  molecular mimicry and, 39–40
  self vs. non-self, 28–31
  stress and. *See* Stress
Autoimmune diet, 123–38. *See also* Cooking, functional; Diet, general; Nutrition; *specific recipes*
  about: overview of, 123
  allergens and, 127
  chemicals and, 125–26
  detoxifying meals, 129
  duration of, 138
  gluten-free foods, 124
  GMOs and, 126
  goal of, 124
  how it works, 124–27
  juicing and cleanses, 133–35
  meal plan samples, 285–91
  nature's answers, 127–29
  organic foods and, 125
  perspective on, 149–50
  produce and, 127–28
  specific foods, 130–33
  water, hydration and, 128–29
  Yes and No foods, 135–38
Autoimmune diseases
  about: overview of, 9–10, 11
  conditions, itemized, 16–19
  defined, 12, 16

historical perspective, 14–15
hygiene and, 42–43, 120–22
reversing, 9, 23, 56, 72–74
risk factors, 19–22
treatments worsening condition, 67–69
Autoimmune myocarditis, 16, 50
Autoimmune thrombocytopenic purpura (ATP), 16, 65
Autoimmune thyroid disease, 16, 53, 117
Avocados
  about: ancient myth, 267; benefits of, 130
  Classic Guacamole, 253
  Liquid Salsa, 267
  Mango and Jicama Salad with, 230
  Protein Power Breakfast, 164
  Refreshing Avocado Soup, 215
Ayurvedic medicine, 81, 119, 267

Baked Sweet Potato Cubes, 262
Bananas
  about: buying plantains, 257
  Banana and Cacao Pudding, 252
  Banana and Dates Shake, 263
  Spiced Apples and Bananas Dessert Salad, 232
  Steamed Sweet Plantains, 257
Basil tea, 267
B cells, 13, 14, 22, 36, 40
Beef
  Argentinean Steak Chimichurri for, 200
  Beef with Butternut Squash Stew, 211
  Perfect and Tender Pot Roast, 185
  Protein Power Breakfast, 164
Beets
  about: benefits of, 130–31; oven-roasting, 268; sweetening, 268; using yellow beets, 207, 231
  Beet and Fennel Blood Strengthener (juice), 275
  Beet and Peach Salad, 173
  Beet Soup, 207
  Egglicious Beet Salad, 174
  Red Head, 268
  Roasted Beet Salad, 231

Roasted Root Vegetables Medley, 237
Root Slaw Salad, 225
Sunny California Beet Salad, 171
Super Immune System (juice), 276
Yellow Mayonnaise Beet Slaw, 230
Berries
  Berry-Nutritious Antioxidant Salad, 232
  Cherry Fire Extinguisher, 269
  Digestive Aid (juice), 277
  Kidney Cleanser, 273
  Pure and Natural Cranberry Sauce, 202
  Red Head, 268
Beverages, **265**–69. *See also* Juicing
  Cherry Fire Extinguisher, 269
  Ginger Cooler, 269
  Golden Triangle Milk, 266
  Liquid Salsa, 267
  Red Head, 268
  Spiked Holy Basil Tea, 267
Biphenyls, polychlorinated (PCBs), 42, 52
Bison sirloin tip, 170
Bite-Sized Smoked Salmon Frittatas, 152
Blood Orange and Arugula Salad, 234
Blood sugar
  balancing, 114, 136, 140, 146, 149, 150, 276
  fruit intake and, 136, 149
  gluten-free lifestyle and, 140
  testing, 65
Blueberries. *See* Berries
Boiling vs. roasting, 173
Boswellia serrata (frankincense), 118
Breakfast, **151**–64
  Bite-Sized Smoked Salmon Frittatas, 152
  Breakfast Fried Rice, 161
  Breakfast Zucchini, 240
  Brown Rice Frittata, 164
  Crustless Spinach and Potatoes Quiche, 159
  Farmer's Egg Casserole, 156

Fluffy Yellow Turmeric Scrambled Eggs, 153
The Perfect Breakfast Potatoes, 158
Poached Eggs and Porridge, 163
Protein Power Breakfast, 164
Resistant Starch Porridge, 162
Salvadoran *Huevos Picados con Ejotes* (Green Bean Scramble), 157
Spicy Kale Scramble, 160
Spicy Zucchini Egg Scramble, 154
Sweet Start Breakfast Porridge, 162
Turkey Breakfast Sausages, 155
Broccoli
  about: benefits of, 130–31
  Cheerful Broccoli (juice), 276
  Coconut Cream of Broccoli Soup, 208
Brown rice. *See* Rice
Brussels sprouts, roasted turmeric, 244
Burgers, 168, 190
Butternut squash. *See* Squash

Cabbage
  about: benefits of, 131
  Classic Coleslaw, 233
  Napa Cabbage Stir-Fry, 247
Candida (*Candida albicans*)
  affecting microphage, 33
  antibiotics and, 95
  beneficial vs. fungal, 97–98
  chemokines and, 37
  cleanses/diets, 134–35, 146, 150, 283
  conditions related to, 97–99
  gender and, 98
  gluten and, 104, 125
  hyphal cell wall protein (HWP-1) in, 104, 125
  IL-17 and, 99
  IL-1β, IL-18 and, 100
  inflammation and, 67, 99–100
  matrix metalloproteinases (MMPs) and, 100
  studies on, 95
Canned foods, 144
Capers

Halibut with Olives and Arugula, 179
Olive and Capers Pasta, 180
Carrots
  about: beta-carotene in, 236; purple/white carrots for color, 237
  Carrot Turmeric Soup, 206
  Curly Carrot Strings, 242
  Detox Special (juice), 274
  Infection Fighter (juice), 275
  Roasted Root Vegetables Medley, 237
  Root Slaw Salad, 225
  Shaved Zucchini and Carrots, 243
  Sweet Pepper (juice), 273
  Turmeric and Dill Carrots, 236
  Vegetable and Egg Soup, 218
Casablanca Chicken Skewers, 191
Cauliflower
  about: colors/nutritional properties of, 209
  Cauliflower and Potatoes (*Aloo Gobi*), 177
  Chicken and Cauliflower Stir-Fry, 178
  Roasted Cauliflower and Turmeric Soup, 209
Celery
  about: benefits of, 132; celery root benefits, 241
  Green Beauty/Smoothie (juice), 274
  Infection Fighter (juice), 275
  Parsnip and Celery Root Mash, 241
  Vegetable and Egg Soup, 218
Celiac disease, 17, 43, 64, 112, 124, 125, 140, 141, 142. *See also* Gluten
Cell-mediated response, 13. *See also specific cells*
Cells. *See also specific cell types*
  adaptive/specific response, 13–14, 34–36
  distinguishing self vs. non-self, 28–31
  human self and, 28–29
  immune cell mediators, 36–39
  innate/nonspecific response, 13, 32–34

nonhuman self and, 29–30
self and, 28–30
Ceviche Marinade (*Leche de Tigre*),
204
Changshan, 120
Cheerful Broccoli (juice), 276
Chemicals. *See* Toxins,
environmental
Chemokines, 33, 37, 97, 99, 100, 110
Chemotherapy, 41
Cherries
Cherry Fire Extinguisher, 269
Cherry Lemonade, 279
Digestive Aid (juice), 277
Chicken
about: roasting, 182
Casablanca Chicken Skewers, 191
Chicken and Brown Rice Salad,
223
Chicken and Cauliflower Stir-Fry,
178
Chicken Breasts with Capers, 179
Chicken Fried Rice, 192
Chicken Salad with Apples and
Grapes, 224
Creamy Spaghetti Squash
Vegetarian Pasta with, 194
Harvest Chicken Soup, 172
Hugo's Chicken *Albóndiga* Soup,
212
Hugo's Homemade Chicken
Stock, 197
Indian-Inspired Chicken
Marinade, 198
Indian-Spiced Chicken Tenders,
184
Pollo Verde (Green Chicken), 177
Rosemary and Sage Chicken, 182
Tom Kha Gai Soup (Thai Coconut
Chicken Soup), 217
Turmeric Rice and Chicken, 189
Chinese medicine, 81, 119
Chocolate
Banana and Cacao Pudding, 252
Dates Stuffed with Chocolate
Coconut Butter, 261
Chronic fatigue syndrome, 17, 98
Cilantro

about: benefits of, 132; juices with,
267, 278; meat dishes with, 177,
187
Cilantro Lime Marinade, 198
Jicama Salad with, 228
Mint Chutney with, 200
Citrus
about: benefits of, 132–33
Blood Orange and Arugula Salad,
234
Ceviche Marinade (*Leche de
Tigre*), 204
Cherry Lemonade, 279
Cilantro Lime Marinade, 198
Inflammation Be Gone (juice),
279
Lemon and Pepper Spaghetti
Squash, 248
Lemon-Ginger Salad Dressing, 196
Lemon Pepper Whitefish, 188
Ojai Ginger Orange Salmon, 175
Cleanses, 134–35
Cobalamin (vitamin B$_{12}$), 113
Coconut
about: coconut butter, 261; oil
benefits, 273
Cherry Fire Extinguisher, 269
Coconut Cream of Broccoli Soup,
208
Dates Stuffed with Chocolate
Coconut Butter, 261
Figs with Coconut Cream, 262
Golden Triangle Milk, 266
Red Head, 268
Silky Butternut Squash Soup with
Coconut Cream, 216
Tom Kha Gai Soup (Thai Coconut
Chicken Soup), 217
Coleslaw, 233
Conditions, autoimmune, 16–19
Cooking, functional
about: overview of, 139
boiling vs. roasting, 173
gluten-free, 140–42
low-histamine foods and, 143–45
meal planning and, 148–49
perspective on, 149–50
resistant starches and, 145–46
spice secrets, 146–47
Cranberry sauce, 202

C-reactive protein, 65
Creamy Salmon Salad, 229
Creamy Spaghetti Squash Vegetarian
Pasta, 194
Crohn's disease, 17, 42, 43, 55, 58, 67,
98, 112, 121
Crustless Apple Pie, 258
Crustless Spinach and Potatoes
Quiche, 159
Cucumbers
Cucumber and Green Bean
Salad, 222
Cucumber Mint Soup, 220
Green Beauty, 274
Green Beauty/Smoothie (juice),
274
Curly Carrot Strings, 242
Cytokines (immune cell mediators),
36–39, 97, 99, 100, 114, 118

Dates
Banana and Dates Shake, 263
Dates Stuffed with Chocolate
Coconut Butter, 261
Dehydration, 128
Dendritic cells (DCs), 13, 33–34
Dermatitis, 17, 18, 42, 43
Desserts. *See* Snacks
Dessert salad, 232
Detoxification, 24
Detoxifying meals, 129
Detox Special (juice), 274
Diabetes, 18
artificial sweeteners and, 137
bacteria and, 30
blood sugar balance and, 149
food intake volume and, 137
fungal candida and, 98
genetics and, 20–21
ginseng and, 119
gluten-free and, 140
helminthic therapy and, 42–43
holistic approach, 23–25
juvenile, 17
minerals and, 115–16
MSG and, 56
PFCs and, 51
SAD and, 103
spontaneous remission, 72–73
vitamin A deficiency and, 110

Diagnosis, 59–74. *See also* Testing
about: overview of, 59; what to expect, 22–23
Candida and, 67. *See also* Candida (*Candida albicans*)
challenges of, 22–23, 60–61, 66–67
doctors to see, 60
environmental considerations, 68–69. *See also* Environment, autoimmune disease and; Toxins, environmental
immunology and, 62
medical approach, 23
misdiagnosis and, 22, 60–61, 66–67
misunderstood conditions, 66–67
nutrition and, 63
physiology and, 61–62
psychology and, 63
symptoms and, 69–72
toxicology and, 62
treatments worsening condition and, 67–69
Diet, general. *See also* Gluten; Nutrition
additive precautions, 55–56
allergens and, 24
general guidelines, 24
good-old days, 102–3
gut health and, 102–4
processed foods and, 24, 55–56, 102, 125–26
SAD, 103
Dinner, **181–94**
Casablanca Chicken Skewers, 191
Chicken Fried Rice, 192
Creamy Spaghetti Squash Vegetarian Pasta, 194
Herbes de Provence–Crusted Halibut, 185
Hugo's Carne Asada–Style Flank Steak, 187
Indian-Spiced Chicken Tenders, 184
Lemon Pepper Whitefish, 188
Moroccan-Inspired Sea Bass, 183
Pan-Seared Salmon with Oregano, 186
Perfect and Tender Pot Roast, 185
The Perfect Salmon Burgers, 190
Rosemary and Sage Chicken, 182

Salmon Pockets, 193
Seared Ahi Tuna Steaks, 186
Sizzling Grilled Lamb Chops, 190
Spanish Lamb Steaks, 188
Turmeric Rice and Chicken, 189
Dressings. *See* Sauces and marinades
Drugs, immune response and, 41, 54, 68, 69. *See also* Antibiotics

Eggs
Bite-Sized Smoked Salmon Frittatas, 152
Breakfast Fried Rice, 161
Brown Rice Frittata, 164
Crustless Spinach and Potatoes Quiche, 159
Egglicious Beet Salad, 174
Farmer's Egg Casserole, 156
Fluffy Yellow Turmeric Scrambled Eggs, 153
Poached Eggs and Porridge, 163
Protein Power Breakfast, 164
Salvadoran *Huevos Picados con Ejotes* (Green Bean Scramble), 157
Spiced Egg Salad, 227
Spicy Kale Scramble, 160
Spicy Zucchini Egg Scramble, 154
Tortilla Española (Spanish Omelet), 169
Turmeric Deviled Eggs, 260
Turmeric Mayonnaise, 196
Vegetable and Egg Soup, 218
Endive and Heart of Palm Salad, 234
Ensalada de Jicama (Jicama Salad), 228
Environment, autoimmune disease and, 45–58. *See also* Toxins, environmental
about: overview of, 21, 45–46
defined, 45
diagnosis and, 68–69
epigenetics and, 47–49, 73, 80
genetics vs., 46–49
locations impacting, 57–58
Epigenetics, 47–49, 73, 80
Esophagitis, 17, 99
Estrogen, 19–20, 21–22, 52, 56–57, 66, 112, 131, 282

Farmer's Egg Casserole, 156
Fats, beneficial, 278
Fecal transplants, 121–22
Fennel, in Beet and Fennel Blood Strengthener (juice), 275
Fermented foods, 143–44
Figs with Coconut Cream, 262
Fish and seafood
about: cooking salmon, 229; cooking tuna steaks, 186; fish sauce, 217; raw fish warning, 176
Bite-Sized Smoked Salmon Frittatas, 152
Ceviche Marinade (*Leche de Tigre*), 204
Creamy Salmon Salad, 229
Halibut with Olives and Arugula, 179
Herbes de Provence–Crusted Halibut, 185
Lemon Pepper Whitefish, 188
Moroccan-Inspired Sea Bass, 183
Ojai Ginger Orange Salmon, 175
Pan-Seared Salmon with Oregano, 186
The Perfect Salmon Burgers, 190
Peruvian Ceviche, 176
Russian Salmon Soup, 214
Salmon Pockets, 193
Seared Ahi Tuna Steaks, 186
Whitefish Soup, 213
Fish oils, 114–15
Fleming, Alexander, 92, 93
Fluffy Yellow Turmeric Scrambled Eggs, 153
Folic acid (vitamin B_9), 113–14
Food. *See* Autoimmune diet; Diet, general; Nutrition
Frankincense (*Boswellia serrata*), 118
Frittatas, 152, 164
Fruit. *See also specific fruit*
autoimmune diet and, 127–28
detoxifying meals with, 129

Garam masala, 184
Garlic
Infection Fighter (juice), 275
Sautéed Green Beans with Fresh Garlic, 238

Sautéed Mushrooms with Garlic, 249
Genetically modified foods (GMOs), 126
Genetics
    autoimmune diseases and, 20–21, 47
    environment vs., 46–49
    epigenetics and, 47–49, 73, 80
    Human Genome Project, 47
    of nonhuman to human cells, 29
Ginger, 118
    about: power and taste of, 272
    Detox Special (juice), 274
    Ginger Cooler, 269
    Ginger Turmeric Potato Salad, 226
    Inflammation Be Gone (juice), 279
    Lemon-Ginger Salad Dressing, 196
    Ojai Ginger Orange Salmon, 175
    Spicy Ginger Charmer (juice or smoothie), 278
    Sweet and Spicy (juice), 272
    Watermelon and Ginger Ice Cubes, 261
Ginseng, 119
Glomerulonephritis, 17, 65
Gluten
    candida and, 104, 125
    cooking without, 140–42
    dining guides for gluten-free, 283–84
    foods without, 124, 140–42
    hidden sources, 141–42
    inflammation from, 103–4
    rise in sensitivity to, 103–4
    testing for, 284
GMOs, 126
Gold, 65
Golden Triangle Milk, 266
Grapes
    Chicken Salad with Apples and Grapes, 224
    Fine and Dandy-lion (juice), 277
    Kidney Cleanser, 273
Green beans
    Cucumber and Green Bean Salad, 222

Salvadoran *Huevos Picados con Ejotes* (Green Bean Scramble), 157
    Sautéed Green Beans with Fresh Garlic, 238
Green Beauty (juice or smoothie), 274
Guacamole, 253
Gut health
    acid reflux, HCL levels and, 61–62
    American Gut Project, 101, 102–3, 283
    antibiotics and, 58, 96–97
    candida and. *See* Candida (*Candida albicans*)
    as "densest ecosystem," 30
    diet and, 102–4
    lifestyle and, 104
    maintaining, 101–4
    microbes and, 30, 91, 101

Halibut with Olives and Arugula, 179
Harvest Chicken Soup, 172
Hashimoto's disease, 17, 116
HCL levels, 61–62
Healing, 75–89. *See also* Herbs; Natural solutions; Treatments; Vitamins and minerals
    about: keys to, 75
    complexity of body and, 76
    holistic approach, 78
    medical approach, 77
    meditation and, 85–86, 87
    mind-body connection and, 81–84
    mindfulness and, 85–86
    nocebo effect and, 83–84
    physical body and, 77–78
    placebo effect and, 82–83
    prayer and, 84–85
    psychological, 78–81
    psychotherapy and, 79–81
    segmentation, dissociation and, 76
    somatic experiencing (SE) and, 87–88, 89
    spontaneous remission, 72–74
    stress reduction for. *See* Stress reduction
    symptoms of, 71–72

tension and trauma release exercises (TRE) and, 88–89
    wholeness of body and, 76
Heart of palm and endive salad, 234
Helminthic therapy, 42–43, 121
Herbes de Provence–Crusted Bison Sirloin Tip, 170
Herbes de Provence–Crusted Halibut, 185
Herbs, 117–20
    andrographis (*Andrographis paniculata*), 117–18
    basil, 267
    chang shan, 120
    cilantro, 132
    frankincense (*Boswellia serrata*), 118
    ginger, 118
    ginseng, 119
    rosemary, 119
    spices and, autoimmune diet and, 128, 146–47
    turmeric, 119–20
Histamines, 143–45
History, of autoimmune diseases, 14–15
Holistic approach, 23–25, 78
Holy basil tea, 267
Homocysteine, testing for, 65
Hormone testing, 66
Hugo's Carne Asada–Style Flank Steak, 187
Hugo's Chicken *Albóndiga* Soup, 212
Hugo's Homemade Chicken Stock, 197
Humoral response, 14
Hydration, 128–29
Hygiene, autoimmune diseases and, 120–22
    fecal transplants and, 121–22
    hygiene hypothesis, 120–21
    hygiene hypothesis and, 42
    worm therapy, 42–43, 121

Ice cubes, watermelon and ginger, 261
Idiopathic thrombocytopenic purpura (ITP), 17
IgA, 17, 38
IL-17, 99

IL-1β, IL-18, 100
Immune system
  about: overview of functioning,
    31–32
  B cells and, 13, 14, 22, 36, 40
  cell-mediated response, 13
  complexity of, 12
  evolving understanding of, 12
  functions of, 12
  humoral response, 14
  nonspecific (innate) responses,
    13, 32–34
  planetary elements and, 14
  specific (adaptive) responses,
    13–14, 34–36
  T cells and, 13, 35–36
  toolbox of, 31–39
Immunoglobulins (Ig), 14, 38–39, 64.
  See also Antibodies
Indian-Inspired Chicken Marinade,
  198
Indian-Spiced Chicken Tenders, 184
Infection Fighter (juice), 275
Inflammation
  candida and, 67, 99–100
  gluten and, 103–4
  IL-17 and, 99
  IL-1β, IL-18 and, 100
  as symptom of disease, 71
  as symptom of healing, 71–72
Inflammation Be Gone (juice), 279
Innate response. See Nonspecific
  immunity
Interleukins, 37, 43, 99, 100
Interstitial cystitis, 17, 98, 99
Iodine, 116–17, 131

Jalapeño relish, 202
Jicama
  about, 225
  Ensalada de Jicama (Jicama
    Salad), 228
  L.A. Streets Fruit Salad, 259
  Mango and Jicama Salad, 230
  Raw Jicama Fries, 253
  Root Slaw Salad, 225
Juicing, **271**–80
  about: benefits of, 133–34
  Beet and Fennel Blood
    Strengthener, 275

Cheerful Broccoli, 276
Cherry Lemonade, 279
Detox Special (juice), 274
Digestive Aid, 277
Fine and Dandy-lion, 277
Green Beauty/Smoothie, 274
Infection Fighter, 275
Inflammation Be Gone, 279
Kidney Cleanser, 273
Spicy Ginger Charmer, 278
Spicy Peppermint Shot, 280
Super Immune System, 276
Sweet and Spicy, 272
Sweet Pepper, 273
The Turmeric Original, 272

Kalamata Olive Spread, 203
Kale
  about: benefits of, 132–33
  Green Beauty/Smoothie (juice),
    274
  Kidney Cleanser, 273
  Spicy Kale Scramble, 160
  Turmeric-Spiced Kale Chips, 254
Kawasaki disease, 17
Kidney Cleanser, 273
Killer Jalapeño Relish, 202
Kiwifruit, in Fine and Dandy-lion
  (juice), 277

Lamb
  Lamb Marinade, 199
  Sizzling Grilled Lamb Chops, 190
  Spanish Lamb Steaks, 188
L.A. Streets Fruit Salad, 259
Leche de Tigre (Ceviche Marinade),
  204
Lemons and limes. See Citrus
Lifestyle, 104
Lipopolysaccharides (LPS), 95–97.
  See also Candida (Candida
  albicans)
Liquid Salsa, 267
Low-histamine foods, 143–45
Lunch, **165**–80
  Beet and Peach Salad, 173
  Cauliflower and Potatoes (Aloo
    Gobi), 177
  Chicken and Cauliflower Stir-Fry,
    178

Chicken Breasts with Capers, 179
Egglicious Beet Salad, 174
Halibut with Olives and Arugula,
  179
Harvest Chicken Soup, 172
Herbes de Provence–Crusted
  Bison Sirloin Tip, 170
Mediterranean Turkey Burger, 168
Ojai Ginger Orange Salmon, 175
Olive and Capers Pasta, 180
Peruvian Ceviche, 176
Pollo Verde (Green Chicken), 177
Resistant Starch Brown Rice, 166
Resistant Starch Brown Rice
  Pasta, 167
Resistant Starch Potatoes, 168
Sunny California Beet Salad, 171
Tortilla Española (Spanish
  Omelet), 169
Lupus, 15, 17, 20, 21, 50, 57, 58, 66, 81,
  98, 110, 126

Macrophages, 13, 32–33, 34
Magnesium, 116
Mango
  Berry-Nutritious Antioxidant
    Salad, 232
  L.A. Streets Fruit Salad, 259
  Mango and Jicama Salad, 230
  Mango Sorbet, 255
Marinades. See Sauces and
  marinades
Matrix metalloproteinases (MMPs),
  100
Mayonnaise, turmeric, 196
Meal planning, 148–49
Meal plan samples, 285–91
Mediators, immune cell, 36–39
Medical approach, 23, 77
Medication, autoimmune diseases
  and, 41, 54, 68, 69. See also
  Antibiotics
Meditation/mindfulness, 85–86, 87,
  104
Mediterranean Turkey Burger, 168
Mercury, 50, 65
Metals, heavy, 42, 50, 65
Microbes
  antibiotics and, 91, 93
  B vitamins and, 111

"good" vs. "bad," 30

gut health and, 30, 91, 101

helminthic therapy and, 42–43

humoral response to, 14

hygiene and, 120–21

IL-1β, IL-18 and, 100

immune system protecting
   against, 12, 14

immune system relationship with,
   30

importance to health, 30

lifestyle and, 104

MMPs and, 100

nonhuman self and, 29–30

non-self and, 30–31

Milk, golden triangle, 266

Milk alternatives, 156

Mind-body connection, 81–84. See
  also Healing

Mindfulness, 85–86

Minerals. See Vitamins and minerals

Mint

   Cucumber Mint Soup, 220

   Mint and Watermelon Salad, 225

   Mint Chutney, 200

   Spicy Peppermint Shot, 280

MMPs (matrix metalloproteinases),
   100

Molecular mimicry, 39–40

Moroccan-Inspired Sea Bass, 183

Multiple sclerosis

   alpha lipoic acid (ALA) and, 114

   chang shan and, 121

   fungal candida and, 98

   genetics and, 20, 21

   gluten and, 67, 103, 124, 140

   helminthic therapy and, 42–43

   mindfulness and, 86

   nutrition and, 63

   processed foods and, 55

   rosemary and, 120

   vitamin B_{12} and, 113

   vitamin D and, 109

Mushrooms

   about: cleaning, 223

   Chicken and Brown Rice Salad,
     223

   Sautéed Mushrooms and Spinach,
     250

   Sautéed Mushrooms with Garlic,
     249

   Tom Kha Gai Soup (Thai Coconut
     Chicken Soup), 217

NAD+, 23

Napa Cabbage Stir-Fry, 247

Naphthalenes, polychlorinated
   (PCNs), 52

Natural killer (NK) cells, 34

Natural solutions, 105–22. See also
  Herbs; Vitamins and minerals

   about: overview of, 105

   alpha lipoic acid (ALA), 114

   fecal transplants, 121–22

   fish oils, 114–15

   hygiene hypothesis and, 120–22

   worm therapy, 42–43, 121

Neuropathies, 16, 17, 18, 51

Neutrophils, 13, 33, 37

Niacin (vitamin B_3), 112

No and Yes foods, 135–38

Nocebo effect, 83–84

Non-GMO Project, 126

Nonhuman self, 28–29

Nonspecific immunity, 13, 32–34

Nutrition

   about: overview of, 24

   deficiency, autoimmune diseases
     and, 41

   diagnosis and, 63

   meal plan samples, 285–91

   supplements. See Vitamins and
     minerals

   testing for deficiencies, 66

Ojai Ginger Orange Salmon, 175

Olives

   Kalamata Olive Spread, 203

   Olive and Capers Pasta, 180

Omega-3 fatty acids, 114–15

Onions

   Pan-Fried Onions with Fresh
     Thyme, 246

   Super Immune System (juice),
     276

Organic foods, 125

Organochlorine pesticides (OCs),
   51–52

PAHs (polycyclic aromatic
   hydrocarbons), 42, 51

Pan-Fried Onions with Fresh Thyme,
   246

Pan-Seared Salmon with Oregano,
   186

Parsnips

   Parsnip and Celery Root Mash,
     241

   Parsnip and Turmeric Soup, 219

   Roasted Root Vegetables Medley,
     237

   Silky Parsnip Mash, 239

Pasta and pasta substitutes

   Creamy Spaghetti Squash
     Vegetarian Pasta, 194

   Lemon and Pepper Spaghetti
     Squash, 248

   Olive and Capers Pasta, 180

   Resistant Starch Brown Rice
     Pasta, 167

Pathogens, 14, 33, 39–40, 100, 104

PBDEs (polybrominated diphenyl
   ethers), 53

PCBs (polychlorinated biphenyls),
   42, 52

PCNs (polychlorinated
   naphthalenes), 52

Peaches, in Beet and Peach Salad,
   173

Pears

   Green Beauty/Smoothie (juice),
     274

   Spiced Poached Pears, 256

   Sweet and Spicy (juice), 272

Pemphigus, 15, 18

Peppers

   Killer Jalapeño Relish, 202

   Lemon and Pepper Spaghetti
     Squash, 248

   Sweet Pepper (juice), 273

Perfect and Tender Pot Roast, 185

Perfect Breakfast Potatoes, 158

Perfect Salmon Burgers, 190

Peruvian Ceviche, 176

Pesticides, organochlorine (OCs),
   51–52

Pets, autoimmune diseases in, 15

PFCs (polyfluorinated compounds),
   51

Pineapple
    Kidney Cleanser, 273
    Liquid Salsa, 267
Placebo effect, 82–83
Planning meals, 148–49
Plans, meal, 285–91
Plantains, steamed sweet, 257
Poached Eggs and Porridge, 163
Pollo Verde (Green Chicken), 177
Polybrominated diphenyl ethers
    (PBDEs), 53
Polychlorinated biphenyls (PCBs),
    42, 52
Polychlorinated naphthalenes
    (PCNs), 52
Polycyclic aromatic hydrocarbons
    (PAHs), 42, 51
Polyfluorinated compounds (PFCs),
    51
Porridge, 162, 163
Potatoes
    about: red, 226; as thickener, 208,
        219; varieties of, 158, 226
    Cauliflower and Potatoes (Aloo
        Gobi), 177
    Crustless Spinach and Potatoes
        Quiche, 159
    Ginger Turmeric Potato Salad, 226
    The Perfect Breakfast Potatoes,
        158
    Resistant Starch Potatoes, 168
    Tortilla Española (Spanish
        Omelet), 169
Pot roast, 185
Prayer, 84–85, 104
Prebiotics, 145
Pregnancy
    autoimmune diseases and, 20
    dehydration and, 128
    folic acid (vitamin B$_{12}$) and, 113
    microbes and, 30, 101
    nutrition and, 107
    toxins and, 53
    vitamin E and, 109
Processed foods, 24, 55–56, 102,
    125–26
Protein Power Breakfast, 164
Proteins, complement, 37–38
Proteins, C-reactive, 65
Psoriasis, 18, 85, 98, 100, 120

Psychology
    diagnosis and, 63
    healing, body, mind and, 78–81
    nocebo effect and, 83–84
    placebo effect and, 82–83
    psychotherapy and, 79–81
Psychotherapy, 79–81
Pumpkin Spice Applesauce, 201
Pure and Natural Cranberry Sauce,
    202
Pyridoxine (vitamin B$_6$), 112

Raspberries. See Berries
Raw Jicama Fries, 253
Refreshing Avocado Soup, 215
Relishes. See Sauces and marinades
Remission, spontaneous, 72–74
Resistant Starch Brown Rice, 166
Resistant Starch Brown Rice Pasta,
    167
Resistant Starch Porridge, 162
Resistant Starch Potatoes, 168
Resistant starches, 145–46
Resources, 281–84
Reversing autoimmune diseases, 9,
    23, 56, 72–74
Rheumatic fever, 18, 39
Rheumatoid arthritis (RA)
    antibiotics and, 58
    diagnosis challenges, 67
    fungal candida and, 98
    gender and, 20
    genetics and, 20–21
    gluten-free and, 140
    historical perspective, 15
    pollution, toxins and, 57
    treatments, 65, 112, 114, 118, 119,
        120
    vitamin A deficiency and, 110
    vitamin B$_6$ deficiency and, 112
Riboflavin (vitamin B$_2$), 112
Rice
    about: cooling process and
        resistant starch, 166, 167
    Breakfast Fried Rice, 161
    Brown Rice Frittata, 164
    Chicken and Brown Rice Salad,
        223
    Chicken Fried Rice, 192

Crustless Spinach and Potatoes
    Quiche (variation), 159
Resistant Starch Brown Rice, 166
Resistant Starch Brown Rice
    Pasta, 167
Resistant Starch Porridge, 162
Turmeric Rice and Chicken, 189
Risk factors, 19–22. See also specific
    risk factors
Roasted Beet Salad, 231
Roasted Cauliflower and Turmeric
    Soup, 209
Roasted Root Vegetables Medley, 237
Roasted Turmeric Brussels Sprouts,
    244
Roasting vs. boiling, 173
Root Slaw Salad, 225
Rosemary, 119
Rosemary and Sage Chicken, 182
Russian Salmon Soup, 214

SAD (Standard American Diet), 103
Salad dressings. See Sauces and
    marinades
Salads, 221–34
    Asparagus Salad, 233
    Beet and Peach Salad, 173
    Berry-Nutritious Antioxidant
        Salad, 232
    Blood Orange and Arugula Salad,
        234
    Chicken and Brown Rice Salad,
        223
    Chicken Salad with Apples and
        Grapes, 224
    Classic Coleslaw, 233
    Creamy Salmon Salad, 229
    Cucumber and Green Bean
        Salad, 222
    Egglicious Beet Salad, 174
    Endive and Heart of Palm Salad,
        234
    Ensalada de Jicama (Jicama
        Salad), 228
    Ginger Turmeric Potato Salad, 226
    L.A. Streets Fruit Salad, 259
    Mango and Jicama Salad, 230
    Mint and Watermelon Salad, 225
    Roasted Beet Salad, 231
    Root Slaw Salad, 225

Spiced Apples and Bananas Dessert Salad, 232
Spiced Egg Salad, 227
Sunny California Beet Salad, 171
Yellow Mayonnaise Beet Slaw, 230
Salmon. *See* Fish and seafood
Salvadoran *Huevos Picados con Ejotes* (Green Bean Scramble), 157
Sauces and marinades, **195**–204
    about: fish sauce, 217; homemade mayonnaise, 227
    Argentinean Steak Chimichurri, 200
    Asian Marinade, 203
    Ceviche Marinade (*Leche de Tigre*), 204
    Cilantro Lime Marinade, 198
    Hugo's Homemade Chicken Stock, 197
    Indian-Inspired Chicken Marinade, 198
    Kalamata Olive Spread, 203
    Killer Jalapeño Relish, 202
    Lamb Marinade, 199
    Lemon-Ginger Salad Dressing, 196
    Mint Chutney, 200
    Pumpkin Spice Applesauce, 201
    Pure and Natural Cranberry Sauce, 202
    South of the Border Aioli, 199
    Turmeric Mayonnaise, 196
Saunas, 24
Sausage, turkey breakfast, 155
Sautéed Green Beans with Fresh Garlic, 238
Sautéed Mushrooms and Spinach, 250
Sautéed Mushrooms with Garlic, 249
Scleroderma, 18, 98
Seared Ahi Tuna Steaks, 186
Selenium, 116, 117
Self
    body's cells and, 28
    human, 28–29
    immune system function for, 28
    nonhuman, 29–30
Shaved Zucchini and Carrots, 243
Silky Butternut Squash Soup with Coconut Cream, 216
Silky Parsnip Mash, 239

Sizzling Grilled Lamb Chops, 190
Skewers, chicken, 191
Smoked meats, 144
Snacks, **251**–63
    Baked Sweet Potato Cubes, 262
    Banana and Cacao Pudding, 252
    Banana and Dates Shake, 263
    Classic Guacamole, 253
    Crustless Apple Pie, 258
    Dates Stuffed with Chocolate Coconut Butter, 261
    Figs with Coconut Cream, 262
    L.A. Streets Fruit Salad, 259
    Mango Sorbet, 255
    Raw Jicama Fries, 253
    Spiced Poached Pears, 256
    Steamed Sweet Plantains, 257
    Turmeric Deviled Eggs, 260
    Turmeric-Spiced Kale Chips, 254
    Watermelon and Ginger Ice Cubes, 261
Somatic experiencing (SE), 87–88, 89
Soups and stews, **205**–20
    about: thickening agents, 208, 219; turmeric in, 214
    Beef with Butternut Squash Stew, 211
    Beet Soup, 207
    Butternut Squash Soup, 210
    Carrot Turmeric Soup, 206
    Coconut Cream of Broccoli Soup, 208
    Cucumber Mint Soup, 220
    Harvest Chicken Soup, 172
    Hugo's Chicken *Albóndiga* Soup, 212
    Hugo's Homemade Chicken Stock, 197
    Parsnip and Turmeric Soup, 219
    Refreshing Avocado Soup, 215
    Roasted Cauliflower and Turmeric Soup, 209
    Russian Salmon Soup, 214
    Silky Butternut Squash Soup with Coconut Cream, 216
    Tom Kha Gai Soup (Thai Coconut Chicken Soup), 217
    Vegetable and Egg Soup, 218
    Whitefish Soup, 213

South of the Border Aioli, 199
Spanish Lamb Steaks, 188
Spanish Omelet, 169
Specific immunity, 13–14, 34–36
Spiced Apples and Bananas Dessert Salad, 232
Spiced Egg Salad, 227
Spiced Poached Pears, 256
Spices, 128, 146–47, 184. *See also* Herbs
Spicy Asparagus, 240
Spicy Ginger Charmer (juice or smoothie), 278
Spicy Kale Scramble, 160
Spicy Peppermint Shot, 280
Spicy Zucchini Egg Scramble, 154
Spinach
    Crustless Spinach and Potatoes Quiche, 159
    Sautéed Mushrooms and Spinach, 250
    Sunny California Beet Salad, 171
    Vegetable and Egg Soup, 218
Spleen, 32
Spontaneous remission, 72–74
Squash
    Beef with Butternut Squash Stew, 211
    Breakfast Zucchini, 240
    Butternut Squash Soup, 210
    Creamy Spaghetti Squash Vegetarian Pasta, 194
    Lemon and Pepper Spaghetti Squash, 248
    Shaved Zucchini and Carrots, 243
    Silky Butternut Squash Soup with Coconut Cream, 216
    Spicy Zucchini Egg Scramble, 154
    Squash Blossom Stir-Fry, 245
    Vegetable and Egg Soup, 218
Standard American Diet (SAD), 103
Starches, resistant, 145–46
Statin drugs, 41
Steamed Sweet Plantains, 257
Strawberries. *See* Berries
Stress
    impacting immune system/ causing disease, 25, 40–41, 48, 80, 81–82
    lifestyle and, 104

overshadowing symptoms, 71
resiliency and, 86–87
vitamins, minerals and, 106–7, 108
Stress reduction, 85–89
about: overview of therapies/
techniques, 25
diet for, 138
ginseng for, 119
lifestyle tips for, 104
meditation/mindfulness for,
85–86, 87, 104
somatic experiencing (SE) for,
87–88, 89
tension and trauma release
exercises (TRE) for, 88–89
turmeric for, 120
vitamin C for, 108
Sunny California Beet Salad, 171
Superfoods, about, 277
Super Immune System (juice), 276
Supplements. *See* Vitamins and
minerals
Sweeteners, 137
Sweet potatoes cubes, baked, 262
Symptoms
acute and chronic, 71
diagnosis and, 69–70
of disease, 71
of healing, 71–72
lack of, 71
nonspecific and specific, 70

T cells, 13, 35–36
Tension and trauma release
exercises (TRE), 88–89
Testing
antibody, 22, 64
blood sugar, 65
C-reactive protein, 65
gluten, 284
heavy metals, 65
homocysteine, 65
hormone, 66
immunoglobulin, 64
nutrient, 66
Thai Coconut Chicken Soup (*Tom
Kha Gai* Soup), 217
Thickeners, 208, 219

Thrombocytopenic purpura
(TTP), 16. *See also* Autoimmune
thrombocytopenic purpura (ATP)
Thymus cells. *See* T cells
TNF-alpha, 37, 40, 48, 97
Tom Kha Gai Soup (Thai Coconut
Chicken Soup), 217
Tortilla Española (Spanish Omelet),
169
Toxins, environmental. *See also
specific toxins*
autoimmune diseases and, 41
babies and, 49–50
burden of, 53–56
chemicals, 42, 49–50, 53–54, 62,
69, 126
detoxifying meals and, 129
diagnosis and, 62
food-related, 42
heavy metals, 42, 50
passed from mother to child,
49–50
processed foods and, 55–56
where you live and, 57–58
women and, 56–57
TRE (tension and trauma release
exercises), 88–89
Treatments. *See also* Healing; Herbs;
Natural solutions; Vitamins and
minerals
common medical mistakes, 76
worsening condition, 67–69
Turkey
about: bison vs., 170
Mediterranean Turkey Burger, 168
Turkey Breakfast Sausages, 155
Turmeric
about: adding color with, 214;
benefits of, 119–20; in soups, 214;
stain precaution, 266
Carrot Turmeric Soup, 206
Fluffy Yellow Turmeric Scrambled
Eggs, 153
Ginger Turmeric Potato Salad, 226
Golden Triangle Milk, 266
Inflammation Be Gone (juice),
279
Parsnip and Turmeric Soup, 219
Roasted Cauliflower and
Turmeric Soup, 209

Roasted Turmeric Brussels
Sprouts, 244
Turmeric and Dill Carrots, 236
Turmeric Deviled Eggs, 260
Turmeric Mayonnaise, 196
The Turmeric Original (juice), 272
Turmeric Rice and Chicken, 189
Turmeric-Spiced Kale Chips, 254

Ulcerative colitis, 18, 98, 112, 121

Vegetables, **235**–50. *See also specific
vegetables*
about: autoimmune diet and,
127–28; benefits by type, 130–33;
detoxifying meals with, 129
Breakfast Zucchini, 240
Curly Carrot Strings, 242
Lemon and Pepper Spaghetti
Squash, 248
Napa Cabbage Stir-Fry, 247
Pan-Fried Onions with Fresh
Thyme, 246
Parsnip and Celery Root Mash,
241
Roasted Root Vegetables Medley,
237
Roasted Turmeric Brussels
Sprouts, 244
Sautéed Green Beans with Fresh
Garlic, 238
Sautéed Mushrooms and Spinach,
250
Sautéed Mushrooms with Garlic,
249
Shaved Zucchini and Carrots, 243
Silky Parsnip Mash, 239
Spicy Asparagus, 240
Squash Blossom Stir-Fry, 245
Turmeric and Dill Carrots, 236
Vegetable and Egg Soup, 218
Vitamins and minerals
about: for autoimmune
conditions, 106, 115; B vitamins,
111
calcium, 115–16
iodine, 116–17, 131
magnesium, 116
multivitamin and mineral
formulas, 106–7

selenium, 116, 117
vitamin A/beta-carotene, 41, 110–11, 216, 236, 273
vitamin B_1, 111
vitamin B_2 (riboflavin), 112
vitamin B_3 (niacin), 112
vitamin B_6 (pyridoxine), 112
vitamin B_9 (folic acid), 113–14
vitamin B_{12} (cobalamin), 113
vitamin C, 41, 108, 273
vitamin D, 41, 108–9, 115
vitamin E, 41, 109–10
zinc, 61, 66, 116

Water intake, 128–29
Watermelon
    L.A. Streets Fruit Salad, 259
    Mint and Watermelon Salad, 225
    Watermelon and Ginger Ice
        Cubes, 261
Whitefish. *See* Fish and seafood
Witebsky, Ernst, 16
Women, autoimmune diseases and, 19–20. *See also* Pregnancy
    estrogen and, 19–20, 21–22, 52, 56–57, 66, 112, 131, 282
    toxins and, 56–57
Worm therapy, 42–43, 121

Yellow Mayonnaise Beet Slaw, 230
Yes and No foods, 135–38

Zinc, 61, 66, 116
Zucchini. *See* Squash